Very Best Wishes

Noel.

Memoirs of a Cow Mechanic

GW00976106

A Dream Fulfilled

A Fun Vocation

By Noel Stuart

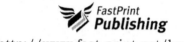

http://www.fast-print.net/bookshop

MEMOIRS OF A COW MECHANIC
Copyright © Noel Stuart 2015

A catalogue record for this book is available from the British Library

ISBN 978-178456-308-0

First published 2015 by
FASTPRINT PUBLISHING
Peterborough, England.

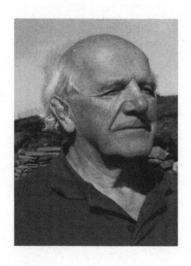

Dedication

AS EVER MY grateful thanks to my parents whose faith and trust helped me through college to achieve my dream and to Margaret, my wife, who has constantly supported me throughout my forty years in practice and has laughed at my funny stories and shared in the joy of my vocation.

To Anne Morgellyn, my tutor, who pointed me in the right direction and to Mike Hales and David Cromey who have so thoroughly checked my errors.

My friend Mike Carter who very skilfully designed the outside cover has special mention.

Of course I must thank my clients and patients who helped me paint the canvas.

Introduction

DEAR FRIENDS! We are in the process of 'coming out'! Previously I have flown under false colours. For those of you who do not already know that Ned Carson, aka Noel Stuart, the handsome, rough and ready veterinary student eventually married Moira, aka Margaret, a devastatingly beautiful young lady. Despite all forecasts she still cares for me after fifty nine years.

As many of you have seem to have enjoyed my first two books, we appear in this third production as Noel and Margaret and I hope to end up where I am now in part of the Celtic fringe, the magical county of Cornwall. It has been a long and arduous road, particularly for Margaret, brought up in the city and dragged away to the country with all its accompanying sights and smells! Despite everything I would be prepared to enjoy all the challenges with her once again.

Memoirs of a Cow Mechanic

A VETERINARY SURGEON

VETERINARY SURGEONS are probably the most important of all horse persons because they not only know all about horses but also about horses that are not feeling very well, and all about horses that are pretending that they are not feeling very well. They also know all about people who are trying to sell horses that are not feeling very well, and people who are trying to buy horses.

Veterinary surgeons are always right and must never be called horse doctors or even 'vets' but only veterinary surgeons or by their Christian names.

This quotation is attributed to Rosie Tesseyman who was one of the most amazing animal handlers I have encountered. She was one of those larger than life people whom everybody loved. Her main asset was a wide open welcome to all and sundry with smiles and laughter. She lived in a rather battered small holding with her group of very contented horses. Her main income appeared to come from teaching children to ride and providing livery. I never could get to the bottom of the origins of all her charges. Her most senior equine character used to wander freely around the premises and had started life in the late 1940s pulling a milk float. He would casually take a bite from any feed bin without detriment. One of Rosies weekly escapades was to collect a load of Brewers Grains from the 'Blue Anchor Pub' in Helston for feeding to her charges. Was this the secret of her success-they were all addicts like we were to her personality.

Chapter One

I RECALL WITH deep affection the enormous 'fluffy' footed draught horses we used to treat on most farms, when it was commonplace to see them pulling ploughs or bringing home loads of turnips or hay to feed the stock. Much of the fodder was run through a chopper to make it suitable for the cattle. Farms were more labour intensive with maybe a dozen cows in the 'shippon' or cowshouse. The cows, each with a name such as Bluebell, Rose or Buttercup, were treated like members of the family as they brought in the income. It was a treat to enter a cow house in the early morning. Each individual would be tied up by the neck in her stall quietly pulling hay from the manger, with a quiet scrunching sound interspersed with the odd burp of satisfaction. The trough in front of them would contain some pieces of groundnut meal mixed with rolled barley to improve the milk yield. Of course this was the era when cows were milked by hand unless you were prepared to invest in machine milking. It was labour intensive but, with experience, the hand muscles soon became attuned and the silence was only broken by the streams of milk squirting into the bucket

In the mind's eye I can still see myself entering the cows' house door with the sun streaming through the cobwebbed windows. The sound of cattle contentedly eating, their bedding and the dung channel covered in golden straw. The all-pervading sweet smell of good hay filled the air and chickens were everywhere. Some would be sitting comfortably on the cow's backs, some pecking around the manger for morsels of barley and the inevitable contented clucking as one more egg was laid in the manger. Behind the milker, head tucked into the udder sat a patient circle of cats quietly awaiting any milk splashed over the side. On those days all was right with the world and I knew that I had found my true vocation.

Driving along the edge of a newly cut field of hay, when the cut grass lies prostrate ready for turning is another great joy as we are enveloped in its aroma. These are some of the joys which are unknown to city dwellers.

The great draught horses, descendants of the war horses of old, had their own problems. One was 'mud fever' caused by standing in wet mud for too long when the heels became painful and inflamed. In those days the main treatment was dressing with gentian violet and lots of TLC in a dry stable. Of course the good horse-keeper avoided this problem with regular attention to the feet. Another condition was 'monday morning leg' where the horse had been fed working rations during the weekend when he was tied in the stable and ended up with lymphangitis in which his leg became immensely swollen and painful. I found this very distressing as horses can show extreme pain by their facial expression.

Many experiences which are ingrained in your psyche are the memories of childhood which are very personal as they intrude into one's small world.

"Now the beauty of the thing when the childher plays is
The terrible wonderful length the days is.
Up you jumps, and out in the sun,
And you fancy the day will never be done;"
From Betsy Lee
by T.E.Brown
Manx Poet and principal of Clifton College

So it was in the beginning. It could be termed a surprise visit. For months my mother had been preparing for the arrival of twins to join her daughter and two sons. Of late there had been some disquiet as there was only one heartbeat. In that era it was the custom to feed the expectant mother and the unborn child that resulted in rather large ladies who seemed to go into purdah in the last third of pregnancy.

It must have been a relief and anticlimax to have only one baby when I weighed in at 14lbs! I feel that it was at this stage that my parents decided to call it a day and settle for four children. Events in the ensuing years proved them to be right.

I didn't realise for years just how fortunate I was to be born in the Isle of Man in 1930. Nostalgia for the "lil island" still clings to my inner core after all these years.

My father was a young and very dedicated medical practitioner. He was handsome and always dressed very smartly in a suit, Homburg hat and spats. This rapidly gained him the name of 'The gentleman doctor'. He was a much respected person in those days when the doctor, parson, lawyer and, dare I say it, the bank manager were looked up to as pillars of the community. He had qualified as a dental surgeon in 1913 and joined up soon afterwards as one of the first qualified dentists in the Royal Navy.

The following four years were momentous and he saw service across the world on HMS Royal Oak and HMS Ramillies. His war culminated with the scuttling of the German fleet at Scapa Flow.

During his visits to Plymouth he met up with a pretty Welsh nurse at Devonport hospital. Their meetings were few and far between when they would rendezvous under the clock at Derry's Cross. It was to be a long and passionate romance as my father, following demobilisation, changed course and went to Trinity College Dublin to study medicine. They met some parental opposition at the thought of an Ulster Presbyterian courting a Welsh Baptist, so they solved the problem and eloped. He must have been regarded as a good catch as I have a photo album full of his discards.

His first employment was as an assistant in a medical practice in Warrington. It must have been somewhat up market as he was chauffeur-driven on his rounds in a Bentley. At the end of a terraced street he would be given a list of houses to visit. Having dealt with those particular patients, the car would be awaiting him at the other end of the street and take him off to his next patients. Life was not easy in that era as the great depression of 1929 was fast approaching.

My mother was very protective of my father as he worked such long hours and thought of little else except his patients. He was a quiet, very private man with a whimsical, naughty sense of humour, which he inherited from his father. When he was not working or stealing my comics, his main hobbies were having a flutter on the horses or football pools.

In contrast, my mother could be the aggressive partner, over-protective of her brood, impetuous and generous to a fault. She was also very demanding of us as teenagers and unwilling to let go of the reins. From November onwards each year she would be very busy in the kitchen making Christmas puddings – more than twenty in some years!

It was an annual ceremony when the baby bath would appear on the kitchen table and pans full of ingredients were poured into it. Then all the children were given the great privilege of taking turns at stirring the pudding ceremoniously. Before cooking, a number of silver coins and trinkets were wrapped up in greaseproof paper and mixing was repeated. This act was greeted with tremendous anticipation by all participants on Christmas day. The mixture was then put into numerous pudding bowls and cooked.

As the festive season drew near my father would depart on his rounds loaded up with Christmas puddings and chickens for his poorer clients with big families, who never could afford to pay his accounts, and would most certainly not have had a 'Merry Christmas'. These were the panel patients who paid a few pence each week into a medical scheme.

In all their married years I only once heard them raise their voices in argument. I never mentioned it until later years that I was upset for days as a result. Theirs was a romance which began in Devonport Hospital in 1916 and ended up with them eloping and getting married in Warrington! I heard that there had once been a heated discussion at home, before my birth, when my mother met several of Dad's medicinal leeches on the staircase. Exit the leeches. Wives can be a bit squeamish!

I had never put much thought into my destiny. Of course you do not contemplate such things when you are four-years-old. At that age I was too busy holding my own against my older siblings, who seemed to regard me as a necessary evil to be led by the hand or blamed for all misdemeanours.

To me the world was full of magic. Early each morning I would be sent outside to feed the gulls on the roof who were impatiently lined up outside trying to lead the queue. I would gaze up in wonder at these greedy, imperious birds squabbling over the crumbs. Little did I realise that this closely reflected human behaviour at the spring sales. To show their gratitude at the end of a free meal the gulls then soar skywards and shower you with bird droppings.

Nanny was rather special to me as she was the ever-present carer. I never knew her true name, although I think that she was called Nan Greer. She was quite young, small and slim with straight cut hair. Many times I have thought that she must have been a saint to have coped with four rather unruly children. She came to the rescue when Ted fell down the stairs, carrying his railway set. A rail was pushed into his mouth, nearly amputating his tongue. She was there staunching the bleeding until my mother and father arrived. She was also the first to hear the crash when I climbed the shelves in the wardrobe, which fell on top of me, pinning me to the ground.

It was always nanny who took us for walks in exciting places like Tromode woods or onto the beach for a picnic. She made us go to church on Sundays to take the pressure off dad whilst he slept in. My siblings and I were brought up in the Isle of Man under the surveillance of nanny and attended the local Presbyterian church each Sunday. I found the whole process very boring except for the week when brother Derek sang a solo "Oh! For the wings of a dove." I was rather envious that I had not been asked.

After nanny left, I was always sent off to Sunday School by myself. I never complained but went off cycling down to the harbour and arrived back just after the end of Sunday school. As it was always before my parents were awake I was never detected. Sorry Mum!

I accepted as normal that many families had a cook, housemaid, chauffeur and a nanny. I didn't even realise that others might feel uncomfortable when I talked of the chauffeur with an unconscious arrogance. Having everything done for me seemed a normal way of life at seven years of age!

We used to rent a cottage, called "The Nest," in Port Erin, on the south of the island, for three months each summer and this is where my first memories arise. Port Erin lies in a horseshoe bay, facing the prevailing SW winds, but protected from their buffeting by a breakwater and harbour. On one side like a sentinel, stood Bradda Head topped by the Milner Tower, whilst on the south Balnahowe rose up and sloped away towards the Calf of Man!

From the front door I could run down the "brooaghs," a steep grassy slope sweeping down towards the promenade, have a quick poke at one of the crabs in the front of the Misses Collisters' shop and dash onto the sands and freedom! Oh, the sheer joy of living! – 'cryin' out' for the happy you feel inside.'

Miss Collister's shop was one of those wooden structures found in many holiday resorts during that era. Now, sadly they have to be passed by planning committees who have not got the vision or eccentricity to be different and settle for a boring mediocrity in order to conform. The shop was a café at one end, and a beach shop and sweet shop at the other end. At the back was the kitchen where teas were made and crabs and lobsters boiled before sale. They also sold bottles of pop which had marbles in the neck to stop the fizz escaping. These were so potent that much of the fizz shot down my nose when I drank from them!

For three long sun-blest months each summer my brother Derek and I would roam barefoot and free as larks. No doubt we were overseen by nanny and my elder brother and sister, but this was not important as they were not included in our world of adventures and make-believe.

Even the opportunist herring gulls who strutted across the beach, in their immaculate grey and white livery, awaiting the fall-out from the numerous picnics, were people friendly. They knew their place and would keep just out of reach of little boys. With their red-flashed beaks and bright eyes they walked back and forth 'kuk-kukking' and defending their allotted patch against all comers.

It was only when I found a dead bird and was deeply absorbed examining it to find why it had died that I realised that it had no teeth. I was also amazed at its light weight which explained why it could drift around so aimlessly in the sky. A possible future as a forensic scientist for seagulls loomed up before me. Unfortunately nanny would not let me take it home for post mortem.

At that time our bad-tempered Pekinese dog had been put to sleep so I had to resort to earthworms and spiders webs for my biological interests. It was inevitable that I should be a carer as my father was a doctor and my mother a nurse. The really formative years were still ahead of me.

I'm sure that heaven is full of beaches like Port Erin. It was a place of great happiness. Down at the harbour there were boats to climb into and mooring ropes to swing on. Fish being unloaded from the "Heather Belle" or just watching Arthur Cregeen repairing his nets. I could even find the odd rotting dogfish for scientific study. They looked just like little sharks with their under slung jaws and mean looking eyes staring coldly into oblivion. What was more they were mighty useful as bait for the crab pots and the fishermen used their rough skins for rubbing down the paintwork on the boats.

There was always something exciting to investigate. Just in front of the Herdman Institute there was a spring that used to gush out of the sand. This was the building site for hundreds of moated sandcastles – until the incoming tide would wash away our dreams. The great excitement was to decorate the castle with anything that came to hand. Razor shells made excellent guns, pointing out to sea, seagull feathers were the banners flying proudly from the turrets whilst stones and limpet shells made up the drawbridge and windows.

Inside would be a vast concourse of people, represented by herring egg cases which look rather like bubble wrap. Then, the next day we would repeat it, knowing that one day we should build a wall high enough to keep out the sea. Another adventure was to walk up the stream, under the promenade, with jam jar and fishing nets to catch lots of little eels. The fact that it also contained sewage was of no concern and only helped to build up our natural resistance to infection.

Farther along the beach Will Watterson had boats for hire. The holiday makers would walk out onto his mobile jetty (a couple of planks set upon wheels) and hordes of half-naked little boys, myself included, were there to push the boats out into the bay and perhaps be rewarded with a penny for our labours.

Sometimes we were allowed to lead the hired donkeys along the beach, whilst hysterical little girls clung desperately onto their saddles, giggling and screaming. We didn't really care if they fell off as long as we could claim our day's reward of an ice cream at the Cosy Nook Cafe at the end of the beach

A most exciting adventure when we were very young was an expedition, chaperoned by nanny, on a fishing trip. Beforehand there would be great activity as we had to go down to the beach digging for lugworm. We would soon be surrounded by gawping holidaymakers' children. "Are you digging for crabs or limpets?" Of course you couldn't expect "townies" to know any better.

A tall black man (the first that I'd ever seen), a student at the marine biological station, stopped one day to ask what kind of fish I hoped to catch. With all the wisdom of a six-year-old I replied, "big cod," which was one of the only fish I knew about. He and I carried on talking and jokingly he asked me if I had ever eaten lugworm, to which I replied, "No mister, but I'll swallow one if you give me sixpence!" When he refused my offer I realised that my first venture into commerce had failed abysmally.

When the big day came, nanny would lead us off towards the Rocky Pool, up the hill towards Collinson's Café, where they sold delicious fruit bon-bons. Then we would head along the cliff path, to Rocky Pool beach. This path led around the various little bays and had strategically-placed seats for old people to rest.

That walk always conjures up a picture of flowers and long grass, interspersed with Veronica and clumps of thrift. The plantain flowers or "soldiers" with their long stems and hard, knotted heads were just waiting for little boys to joust with them, so every journey became a new adventure. This is the only spot in the island that I have seen lizards basking in the warmth of a summer's day. I only ever managed to catch one, which ran off, leaving its tail in my hand.

We spent many hours fishing in the Rocky Pool, which appeared enormous to us, although it seems to have shrunk over the years. Such was our skill that the only fish that we caught were with nets. Shrimps, hermit crabs and bullheads were our main prey although there was a hole under one rock that almost certainly contained a conger eel or a large crab. We never waded too deep lest we were attacked by these denizens of the sea.

In the bay next to Rocky Pool was the Port Erin swimming pool, built into the cliff, and filled with water pumped in from the sea. I never progressed beyond the shallow end as I had not learned to swim. On one memorable day, when I was caught by the inflowing water and carried out of my depth, I saved myself by dog paddling back into the shallows. The pool was the centre of social life for all the young people on a warm day, when our time would be interspersed between the water, lying out sunbathing on the hot rocks, or eating ice creams.

The afternoon air was rent with the screams of the girls and shouts of young lads showing off as they chased them around the pool. One afternoon there was much screaming from the girls (who else!) and one of the Challenor girls in a panic said that she had swum in the deep end and met a shark! With my experience of all things aquatic I guessed that it was probably only a dogfish and she was being all theatrical. Girls were a bit unpredictable!

Even at this stage I was becoming absorbed by animals. I had pestered my parents for a dog or a cat, but I had to be content with wild animals. Imagine my great delight when father brought a little West Highland terrier back from his holiday in Scotland. I walked around with him in my arms for a full twenty-four hours in case he disappeared. Soon we became inseparable companions and involved in each other's games. We sulked together when the world was against us and we stood in the corner together when we (or one of us) had been particularly bad.

Like myself this little dog, christened "Mike", was scruffy and not very often a pristine white in colour. He never really lived up to his kennel name of "Michael of Watten". I got into severe trouble when nanny found that I had painted him green instead of bathing him. I never could understand this as he much preferred being painted to having a bath. For quite a long time my mother was concerned that I always seemed to get bitten when I was told to take Mike for a walk in the garden. The reason, I later learned, was that dogs don't like being carried around the garden by their tail, which was my mode of exercising him!

My father, the good doctor, would not have a cat in the house as "they are always living with fleas and carry disease!" He had never encountered cats at close quarters and realised their powers of seduction. His grandparents had been farmers and cats were essentially kept for vermin control and definitely barn-living creatures. Little did he realise that, in time, he would become "catalysed"!

During our walks up on Bradda Head, the long grass was teeming with insect life, the air would be full of the chirping of grasshoppers and they would leap or fly away in clouds, like chaff before the wind, at our approach. It was a great source of annoyance to me that I could stalk the source of their sound only to have it cease as I drew near. There were butterflies, daddy-long-legs and the very mysterious "cuckoo spit" that all required investigation.

As she lacked the same scientific purpose, nanny was not very keen on all these little creatures being kept in jam jars on the window sill. Of course they all had to be taken apart, after death, to find out how they worked. In one of those strange fits of adult pique, nanny banned a dead mouse and seagull being brought back for post mortem! This particular incident could have been a great loss to science. It used to worry me that I might end up like her when I grew up.

In the spring, the cliffs would be a carpet of sky blue squill and patches of gorse, glowing an irridescent yellow in the sunshine. The gentle popping of the seed pods and delicate coconut scent would fill the otherwise quiet afternoon air. The only other sounds to break the stillness were the peep-peep of oyster catchers on the rocks below or the chirring of choughs as they would fall around the sky above our heads.

I would lie in bed in the morning, watching the blue sky through my jam jar collection, hearing only the gentle lapping of the waves on the shore below and the crying of the gulls as they searched the beach for any scraps left behind by the visitors. Mrs Woodworth next door would be out at the front gate scattering her crumbs and shouting "gulla-gulla" to attract the birds. All was right with the world! Strangely, these two sounds still affect me very deeply.

As boys we would spend many hours in the aquarium at the Marine Biological Station, which was associated with Liverpool University. At the entrance there was a small cashier's window set up so high that even the cashier had to look upwards when collecting the entry fee. Being small, we exploited this situation by following a large person into the entry. As the cashier looked upwards and her vision was blocked, we bent double and scuttled in without paying.

We spent hours inside studying the various displays, but mostly the fish – an ever changing view of underwater life! The tanks were full of perpetual motion as cod and calig (pollack) drifted around in their own little dream world. Coalfish, known locally as 'bloggan' or "shitties", shared tanks with whiting, ballan and cuckoo wrasse, whilst the twitching feelers of lobsters and crayfish wafted out of crevasses in the rock. The tanks containing octopus were always interesting, particularly if they moved. They changed colour so rapidly, suddenly going very pale as if they were about to faint.

The larger tanks were always occupied by conger eels and our ambition was to see one that was so big that it couldn't turn around. Often they were up to four or five feet in length and would gracefully glide in and out of holes in the rock and lie there with mouths agape as if awaiting a passing victim. A thrill of horror would run through us as we realised that these were small compared to the eel in the Rocky Pool!

There was one shallow, open tank containing shrimps, hermit crabs and delicate sea anemones whose tentacles waved gently back and forth in the recirculating water. Some of the bigger boys said that if you dropped a halfpenny into an anemone they would, after a few days, divide into two anemones. The scientific desire to experiment was always overcome by the very real fact that we might actually lose our money!

In another room were a series of tanks for growing on plaice and lobster fry for possible restocking purposes. I grew up as one of those learned little guys who knew that plaice started off swimming vertically like other fish and that lobsters were free swimming in their early stages. The die was cast at this early stage, viz. even bad little boys like myself could metamorphose into something better as life went on.

As we left the aquarium there was a mad rush down to the breakwater to watch people fishing and maybe acquire a couple to take home for tea. We could look over the edge and watch ballan swimming around the rocks or even a large conger insinuating his devious passage through the seaweed. We once saw a jellyfish stranded on the rocks that must have been three feet in diameter. Wow! Then off home for tea with a short call at the lifeboat house in case they were giving away any free badges.

On occasion boys, by the very nature of the beast, have to rebel, not that we were under much discipline as my mother was very strongly against physical punishment. Apart from throwing a stone at a charabanc window (I must confess that it was me and I'm awfully sorry Mr coach owner!) and pinching a packet of fruit gums from Miss Collister's shop, for a dare, I felt that I lived a fairly impeccable life. Mind you, I could spit farther and more accurately than any of my friends, which gave me some social standing.

If I was ever bored I used to wait for the arrival of "Ginny" the milk lady. She would arrive each day with a horse pulling a brightly painted milk float. The small bay mare, "Anna" liked nothing better than to be fussed over by little boys with sugar lumps in their hands. All the brasses on her harness were kept shining brightly to complement the float. On the float was the most enormous copper milk churn, bound in gleaming brass and from the base projected a large brass tap overhanging the rear. Hanging beside the churn were four glistening jugs. Two pint size and two of a quart capacity.

Imagine how important I felt at being allowed to walk along the road beside the float as Ginnie's helper. To be able to turn the large shiny tap and fill up the copper jug and pour the creamy milk into the householder's own jug was a source of great joy. In case she was delayed a long time Ginny always carried a net full of hay in the float for Anna, her team mate.

One of my vivid memories of a pre-war summer was when the owner of the "Heather Belle", Mr Woodworth and his son Peter, invited me out for a short trip. This involved sailing around to the most southerly tip of the Isle of Man where we hove to at slack water (between the tides), in "The Sound", a treacherous piece of water with a tidal rip running between the mainland and the Calf of Man.

There were several cows, with rope halters on, secured near the water's edge. They were then tied to a rope trailing from the stern of the "Heather Belle" and towed across the Sound to Cow Landing on the Calf of Man where they joined the resident cattle herd. I was amazed that they didn't sink but of course I was too young to know that each one had a built in 50-gallon flotation bag in the shape of the paunch or first stomach.

Life was so exciting as information flowed into my brain that I realised that I did not consider formal education as being very necessary. Dad was always the intellectual family member and fully absorbed in his work. It never occurred to me that mum might be overlooking our development.

Initially we all went to St Francis High School, the 'Red School', run by the Misses Chapell and Stansfield. It was reported to be ideal for the children of the upper middle class. I think that I must have been an abject failure. All that I can recall is making patterned baskets where we stitched wool into a canvas frame and dancing around the room holding hands with a 'soppy' girl to the accompaniment of a piano. When it was suggested that I learned to play the piano I dug my toes in – it was all cissy stuff – no earthworms or beetles to play with!

My next school was with Mrs Edwards, the wife of a sea captain, who lived in Little Switzerland and gave private tuition. Each morning, sister Jane and I would cycle (I was on a tricycle) across Douglas to school. Whilst we awaited Mrs Edwards' arrival in the room she gave us the very practical chore of folding newspaper to use as firelights (I have a PhD in this skill). We were then given spelling and maths all day. She did instil spelling into me. Maths was a bit different until one day she threw her pen at me in sheer frustration.

I must confess that this adventure did not continue for long. Mum, who was incapable of instructing me, then sent me to the Collegiate school run by the Rev Bert Reid and his sisters.

This was a much more enjoyable situation with a few dozen boys and girls. I was slowly beginning to read at eight years old and spent many hours at home absorbed in books –

including a pirated copy of 'Married Love' by Dr Marie Stopes.

Eventually I was sent to Douglas High School with Derek despite my mother's fears that we might mix with common boys who swore and had snotty noses. However all was well because I knew most of the swear words and wiped my nose on my sleeve. I was not really destined for genteel circles!

Chapter Two

DURING MY YOUNGER days I had a recurrent dream in which I saw myself as a horse being ridden by my sister, two brothers and myself – as if we were off to Widdecombe Fair! I never did have the dream analysed but assumed that it was a resentment of the fact that I was the youngest and always being put upon by my elders. Come to think of it, most of my clothes were "hand me downs" from my brothers. Even when we played charades I always had the "cissy" parts. I remember being sat in the middle of a car inner tube and being told that I was a goldfish in a pond and to "shut up" as fish only went 'glub-glub' or something.

Even in those early years Ted always tried to be the "pack leader". This was part of his make-up, as the second child, which stood him in good stead in later years when his drive made him very successful in his chosen profession. He was very dominant and used to bully Cecile (Jane) and the gentle Derek to get his own way.

At this stage I would become very aggressive, put down my head and, with arms flailing, charge at him like a rather chubby battering ram to hit him in the solar plexus. Even Derek, "the dreamer", became so incensed with him one day when he was attacking Cecile, that he swung his camera case in the air and caught Ted a mighty clout on the head.

The advantage of a larger family, over an only child, is that the problems become diluted and generally we got on very well together. Derek and I were very close, shared many of our secrets, and enjoyed each other's company.

We were extremely fortunate when we were at 'Inst' as we could visit my aunt 'Adden' and grandparents who had a grand house and garage at Hanover Place – now, sadly, turned into a supermarket. Some of the happiest days of my life were spent there.

I was not naturally aggressive, unless I was fighting for a cause: c.f. Don Quixote, when I could go off in a wild fury. I feel that I was born with a strong sense of fairness. After one such occasion I told my grandmother that I had previously hit Ted in the leg with a very blunt axe in one of my tempers. Gran's lips tightened into a severe line as she looked straight at me through her gold rimmed spectacles and gently and quietly she said, "You know, my dear, that was very silly as it might have been serious. Always remember that losing your temper is a sign of weakness of character when you cannot think straight!" Under this admonition from an eighty-four-year-old gran most twelve-year-olds would start to wilt. As my eyes filled and my lip trembled she relented and said, "Now come along with me and don't be upset. Let's see if I have any biscuits in my pantry"

A visit to gran's pantry held great magic and always filled me full of awe. It was large and airy with red tiles on the floor, which helped to keep it cool. It didn't smell of lavender like my grandmother, but had its own never-to-be-forgotten aroma. On rows of shelving stood all the family china (except of course the chinese tea set, displayed in a glass fronted cabinet in the drawing room), the georgian silver tea set, doyleys and tablemats.

All the stores for the kitchen such as bags of flour, baking soda and jars of dried fruit were neatly arranged around the walls alongside the tea and sugar. Behind the door, rows of home-made jam and marmalade stood beside tins containing biscuits and home-made cakes prepared for Sunday tea. This spot was our haven when we needed succour.

Those few words from my grandmother, concurrent with the onset of puberty, started me off on a period of self-examination in which I learned to control my reactions. This lesson was reinforced in physics two years later where

Newton's Law of Motion states that "Action and Reaction are equal and opposite". How true this is in human nature where aggression engenders a similar response.

I had a similar response from gran, when one day I said "damned thing!" after I hit my finger with a hammer. Once again she fixed me with her penetrating, bespectacled stare and said, "You know, my dear, that is not a nice word to say. Swear words are offensive to those who hear them and a sign of a lack of education and self-control." Once again I was in trouble from my dear old Gran, but the message did sink in. I can't recall whether it warranted a visit to the biscuit tin in her pantry.

Chapter Three

NINETEEN-THIRTY-NINE was a very dramatic year in my life and, but for the dedication of my family, I should have been a statistic. Catching my first trout on rod and line was to shape my future. We also acquired a three-storeyed house on Bradda, in Port Erin, called "Thie Cronk" and I contracted pneumonia and tuberculosis!

I did make a definite mistake at the outbreak of war when food rationing was imposed. In a fit of mischief I mixed sugar, salt and pepper together on the breakfast table. It came as quite a shock to find that my dad was not amused and consequently I spent a week without sugar on my cornflakes as I didn't like pepper. Life can become very hard!

That first summer at "Thie Cronk" was idyllic in many ways. The house was overlooking Port Erin bay, yet far enough from the main road for us to play in safety. As we had a garage at the back of the house, my caring siblings decided that, as I was the smallest, I could help them with an interesting experiment. We all climbed onto the garage roof. I had cushions tied onto me, front and back. I was then handed an open umbrella, as a parachute, and they pushed me over the edge. Unfortunately, Mary Poppins had not been invented and I landed rather hard, cushioned by layers of fat, shaken – but undaunted. Nanny promptly called a halt to the experiment!

It was rather unfair to expect her to manage us in this house as we suddenly realised how much more freedom we now had. There were rumours that the "Black Hand" Gang were going to attack us so we constructed a tree house in a nearby fir tree. Here we could hatch plots and plan to repel all boarders during the assault. It wasn't until many years later that we found out that there never had been a "Black Hand" Gang, only very fertile imaginations. As I climbed down out of our tree one day I stood on a bees nest. Fortunately, I ran away after receiving one sting but my brother who was following was attacked quite severely.

I had noticed a pair of jackdaws who kept going into a chimney pot on top of the house. My compassionate side came to the fore and I felt that they probably had nestlings that could benefit from help. Nanny returned from shopping to find that I had climbed out of the skylight, scrabbled up the roof and was sitting on the ridge tiles, three storeys up, dropping worms into the young birds whilst the parents were attacking me as best they could.

Thinking back on this escapade fills me with horror. There was a severe scolding when I came in from the roof. I suspect that I kicked nanny and called her 'a bugger' (new word!) whereupon she administered a well-deserved beating. I believe that when she later reported this to my mother, who did not believe in corporal punishment, she received notice instead of me getting into trouble. I have felt guilty ever since as she had for many years been a locum mum to all of us. I never fully forgave my mother for this as I regarded her as my 'nan'.

Shortly after this incident I developed TB, as a result of which nanny received a temporary reprieve. I lost six weeks of my life before recovering enough to be aware of my surroundings. Dad and his partner worked night and day to pull me through whilst nanny and my mother took turns in nursing me. The sulpha drugs had just come onto the market and I received so much M&B 693 that, in theory, I should have died from the cure!

I still have vivid memories of this period. Hours spent lying in bed just looking around the bedroom. In front of the fireplace there was a pale blue enamelled electric fire. I could see out of the bedroom windows to a block of flats opposite or the top of the mountain ash in the garden.

Sometimes I would hear the foghorn on foggy nights warning sailors in the bay. During the day I could hear the cries of street vendors outside with their horses and carts – 'fresh 'erring, fresh 'erring.' or the rag and bone man on his round – 'rag 'a bone, rag 'a bone.'

At this time I was drifting in and out of consciousness and several times I found myself looking towards the small window and suddenly it would drift away and become smaller as if viewed through a reverse telescope – strange – was this an end of life experience as I struggled to get air into my flooded lungs? This experience has left me with a claustrophobic sensitivity. It resembled my interpretation of 'Alice through the Looking Glass.

Shortly after my recovery I woke up during the night and saw a cowled figure standing over my bed with a hand held out in blessing. In sheer terror I disappeared under the clothes and didn't reappear until morning. I said nothing for several days until I was questioned by my mother as I was unusually subdued. When the story tumbled out my rather fey mum was not particularly amazed.

"You see," she said, "It was probably the spirit of a kindly monk as this house is built on the site of an ancient monastery. If you are ever frightened and alone just repeat the Lord's Prayer and you will find comfort." This one small piece of advice has stood by me all my life!

My antecedents living in Ulster during the nineteenth century had little problem with belief. They accepted the Garden of Eden, immaculate conception, and reincarnation as factual. Those people who were better educated realised that stories that were repeated over the centuries became blurred around the edges. Despite the aims of love and peace enthroned in most faiths, the interpretation put upon it by mankind has been the source of many wars down the centuries.

As children in the Isle of Man, under the surveillance of nanny, we attended the local Presbyteriasn church each Sunday. I found it quite boring except for the week when brother Derek sang a solo, "Oh for the wings of a Dove" which made me quite envious.

The nice thing about being ill was that I slept in the same room as my parents. I was very impressed one night to see them kneel at their bedside in prayer just like nanny had taught us.

The fact that the war had just started did not influence me greatly at the time. I was sent off to Glen Mooar on the West Coast to recuperate by the sea for three months. I stayed with Mrs Kissack, a widow, who could not have been kinder to a now very thin and pale little boy. She poured food into me in such quantities that I soon put on weight and showed an interest in my surroundings. The only cloud on my horizon was that nanny had left and gone into war work.

Living out in the country was for me an idyllic existence, particularly as the weather was warm and I could run free. There were rabbits to stalk along the hedgerows until I discovered that they were smarter than I was and did not completely trust little boys. There was also a small stream running nearby and I would spend hours just lying on the bank watching the trout and sticklebacks. Lifting up stones in the river I found the larvae of dragonflies and other aquatic creatures. These all ended up in a jam-jar on Mrs Kissack's windowsill along with the daddy-long-legs and earwigs.

Yet another great discovery was that the sex of earwigs could be told by the shape of their fearsome but harmless pincers at their rear end. I had been nipped painlessly by them a couple of times. Why does the male have curved pincers whilst the females had straight? Surely they must be used for mating – hence the difference in shape. I did read a book which suggested that they were for defence or packing the wings away in those that actually had wings.

Isn't life fascinating when you have an enquiring mind, which rapidly becomes filled with a mass of useless information?

Mr Robinson, in the bungalow next door, used to lend me his fishing rod and I would disappear down the stream for hours at a time, only to return triumphantly with my catch for the day, several tiny trout. One day, I was sitting dangling a worm in a pool beneath the waterfall, called "Spooyt Vane", and hoping for great things, when I became distracted by a number of magpies chattering in a thorn bush.

The group increased until eventually there were thirteen in the tree. "One for sorrow, two for joy" -there were too many for the rhyme so I politely said good morning to them for luck, as I had been taught. Why, I thought, were they all gathering together in October – maybe a chapel meeting as they are rather social birds!

Lying in bed half asleep one night I heard a most shrill cry outside, like a baby in distress.

After a couple of minutes the screaming ceased and in the ensuing silence and blackness my imagination ran wild and I felt very frightened and vulnerable. There is nothing more disturbing than the unexplained, so I pulled the blankets over my head, followed my mother's advice and repeated the Lord's Prayer before falling into a fitful sleep.

I discussed it with my friend, Mr Robinson, next day and he had also heard the cry. "You must get used to sounds like that if you want to live in the country," he said reassuringly, "I'm pretty sure that it was a polecat killing a rabbit, which screamed out in fear."

I felt a bit braver after that, although a short while later I was walking through the bracken as it was getting dark when I heard a snuffling, grunting sound in the undergrowth. Armed with a large stick in case I was attacked I gently parted the ferns and found the culprits – a pair of hedgehogs having a territorial dispute!

Chapter Four

WHEN I RETURNED home the war impinged on my life. It had already been under way for a couple of months and I had been insulated from it during my stay in the country.

As a special present I was given a cat for my Christmas present. Of course I was overjoyed and played with it constantly. She was called "Suzie" and rapidly settled down to charm my father who didn't really like cats. Fortunately she was accepted by Mike who thought that all cats were meant to be chased up trees.

I was a very thin boy at this stage after my TB. I cannot recall any of my friends being obese as we led active lives and we were on wartime rations. I can look back now and only have compassion for many of the present-day children who are obese and suffering from fat problems.

My eldest brother and sister were at school in Coleraine, Northern Ireland, under the watchful eye of my aunt and grandparents. The housemaid and chauffeur had both departed to help in the war effort, so that depleted the household to Mona, the cook, and the family.

This meant that those left at home had to carry out the chores that the staff had originally done. Heaving scuttles of coal up three stories twice daily and cleaning grates came as a painful surprise to Derek and me.

Black outs and air raid precautions were the main topics of conversation and air raid practices took place with great regularity. My mother became a superintendent in the Red Cross and spent much of her time lecturing V.A.D.s whilst Derek and I were appointed as cycle orderlies to the local Red Cross station.

This pleasant task involved presenting ourselves at many of the meetings so that all the trainees could practice their bandaging skills upon us. Very rapidly we resembled

Egyptian mummies being fussed over by a squad of demented nurses. The job did have its bonuses however as we had lots of glasses of orange squash and biscuits to eat.

The Isle of Man had no problem in declaring war against Germany at the onset of hostilities as it had forgotten to make the peace after the First World War.

Very soon the island was swarming with members of all the forces as they had training bases on the island. By mid-1940, troops were also brought in to guard the various internment camps that had taken over the hotels and boarding houses in the towns.

The complete towns of Port Erin and Port St Mary were surrounded with barbed wire to contain large numbers of German and Italian women who had freedom inside the wire enclosures and could associate with the local population. From our point of view, despite their incarceration they seemed to have many comforts and appeared to be able to get hold of many foods that we never saw in the shops.

One of the first camps was constructed near the promenade in Ramsey and another in Peel was erected to house known enemy sympathisers.

As we owned a house in the town we had permits to enter Port Erin on holidays. My father's partner had joined the forces so dad had to run a two-man practice by himself for a period, until he sustained a heart attack from too much pressure and brought in another doctor to assist him.

I had seen his evening surgeries go on until eleven p.m. and then he would depart on several calls before returning for supper. This type of pressure was unremitting and it was essential that he found assistance to cope with the extra work in the internment camps, and give himself the time to escape to Port Erin for a few weeks.

Communications were restricted as maybe only half of the homes could afford telephones. Our phone had an ear piece shaped like a trumpet and was suspended from a crook. To get through to the exchange we had to crank a handle before talking to the operator.

My cat Suzie quickly got to work on my father's affections. When he was sitting in the lounge, late in the evening, making up his ledger for the day, the cat would sit on the table and pat his pen each time it passed by.

During the day, Suzie would greet all the patients at the front door, escort them into the waiting room, and try out each person's lap in turn, grading them, no doubt, on a comfort scale. She was quite well known on the terrace as she would accost anyone by rubbing against them, trying out her powers of seduction to drum up business for dad.

Her world was shattered when my father was taken off in the ambulance to the hospital, a mile away, with a mild heart attack. Early next morning, as is their wont, the duty nurse, who was my father's patient, breezed into his room, drew the curtains open and said, "Doctor, there is a cat out here that looks just like your Suzie!"

Indeed, by some telepathic means Suzie and dad had made contact, so she had come over a mile to visit! How did they get in contact? I had no idea but my mind was opened later in life when I realised that my mother and sister had the same unconscious gift. This opened up yet another facet to my investigative mind which I have seen re-enacted many times.

When we did manage to steal a few days in Port Erin we had complete freedom within the confines of the perimeter fence and spent many happy hours fishing and bathing. There was a flat rock below Bradda, which was useful for both fishing and swimming.

Many of the German internees had been brought up in the 'Health and Beauty' culture of pre-war Germany. It was during their sunbathing sessions that it slowly dawned upon me that some of these statuesque ladies, who insisted on naked sunbathing, were made in a different shape to men. I spent a long time asking myself why. It was no use asking adults as they always confused the issue.

I was playing outside the house one day when my attention was caught by a sheep walking up the road with a long string of sorts hanging from its rear end. It was followed by a baaing little lamb. At this stage I knew nothing about afterbirths! Full of excitement and scientific fervour I rushed into the house to ask Mum about this strange phenomenon.

As she was half way through baking a cake she didn't seem to have my enthusiasm to rush up the road to examine the sheep's bottom. Instead I was enrolled as pastry chef whilst we had a long discussion on lambs, placentas and planting seeds, which I found absolutely enthralling. I don't suppose many little boys have their first sex education lessons whilst rolling pastry! I suspect that I spent a long time telling God the facts of life when I said my prayers that night.

Needless to say I spent the next week walking through the fields looking at sheep's bottoms. Lambs and calves started to hold a completely different meaning for me. I often wondered whether they got into trouble as much as I did from my mum.

Back at home in Douglas my brother Derek and I attended the local high school, which meant a walk of one and a half miles each day. This walk always had its fascination as there were several routes that we could take. The most direct journey was along Woodbourne Road where we could scuff through sycamore leaves and "flying angels" in the autumn, or if we went up the back lanes, there was a good opportunity to scrump apples.

Many of the boys came in from the outlying towns by bus or train and had to start off fairly early in the morning. They would often arrive in late so we could slip in with them, unnoticed. Sometimes we got into scrapes with boys from Murray's Road school who would jeer and taunt us, chanting "High School sausages, one or two a penny".

I think that it was a good school at the time although I never seemed to excel at much except perhaps nature study and poetry. In my nature study examinations each term I generally came in the top six.

Any limited success I had was due to one teacher, May Lace, who encouraged us to listen to school radio broadcasts on history and nature study and stimulated my first interest in poetry. The rest of my results were so appalling that I normally finished up about thirty third out of thirty-five in the class.

The Peter Pan factor ruled and I could not understand why people swotted so hard when there were all sorts of other, more interesting, things to fill the day. I was quite skilled at marbles, could preserve a fairly hard "conker" and had a good knowledge of stamps (and countries) and aeroplane recognition. Despite my obvious academic drawbacks, Derek and I produced a weekly newsletter for our class with the help of a "Bulldog" printing kit. It did give us some credit with the teaching staff, but it didn't help our examination results.

On the whole I did not get into too much mischief at school apart from the 1st of April 1943, when I wanted to 'April Fool' one of my friends. This consisted of placing the wastepaper basket on top of the classroom door so that it fell on his head as he entered.

The ploy worked admirably apart from the fact that it was the headmaster, Bill Sykes, who entered the room. He did not take kindly to this jape and there was a lot of humble pie consumed in the head's office that day!

I could never recall my mother appearing at school sports days or at prize-giving as we were not in that league. Her interest in outdoor activities was non-existent and she constantly tried to stop us playing football as the grass was damp. This problem was overcome when Derek (her blue-eyed boy) looked at her one day and with wide-eyed solemnity announced that she need not worry as we had under-pitch heating at the Boys High School.

I could never have got away with it but she accepted it as gospel. By this time I was so keen that the next week I was picked to play. I was the goalie but, lacking positional awareness, I quickly scored a goal against the opposition.

When we got home from school the house would be empty as everyone else would be working or fighting a war! We must have been some of the earlier latchkey children. Derek would go off to do his homework but I would be away playing bicycle polo in one of the side streets. This involved any number of players on bicycles, each armed with a walking stick, and a tennis ball. There were no set rules to the game so it went on for a long time or until a stick went through the spokes and the unfortunate victim retired with a collapsed wheel.

Four or five of us who were friends joined the Sea Scouts at the same time. The camps and outdoor activities kept us fairly involved, particularly when we staged a concert with the Sea Rangers.

It was then that I was smitten with my first true love! This gorgeous creature must have been all of ten-years-old, whilst I had reached a mature eleven. I was fickle enough to abandon her big sister for her undoubted charms. This was just as well as my brother Ted married her big sister twelve years later! I must have been rather like a labrador puppy – full of enthusiasm but tripping over its feet all the time in its enthusiasm. I even took up visiting the public swimming baths every Saturday and learnt to swim, as she would be there with her sisters!

Despite these other activities all the boys would go around together, cycling down to the beach or just wandering around unsupervised. To their credit they did rescue a little boy from drowning in a static water tank on one occasion. Inevitably we became bored and got into mischief when someone threw a stone through a car window and took away the emblem on the car's bonnet. Unfortunately for us the car belonged to a police sergeant, who was not well pleased. Nobody confessed to the crime but it made us all sit back and think more seriously about life after we were questioned by the police. It was a result of circumstances where there was insufficient supervision of children during the war.

On the whole any wickedness was restricted to scrumping my English teacher's pears and throwing snowballs at policemen's helmets, although it could have ended anywhere if left to my own devices.

Derek and I did meet up with a certain amount of disapproval on occasions when we discovered a technique for controlling traffic flow. At that time traffic lights were controlled by rubber pressure pads set into the road. If I jumped onto the pad the green light would turn red, stopping the oncoming traffic and the right angled side road light would turn green.

Derek in turn would jump on the side road rubber pad, which would then turn red against the traffic. There was never any great danger from traffic accidents as there were few cars on the roads. But it was great fun! No wonder people were exasperated by those awful Stuart boys!

My mother had heard that the local public school, King William's College, in Castletown, permitted corporal punishment and so decided that her two youngest children should also be sent to Ireland for their education, notwithstanding the fact that the Irish Sea was alive with U-boats. She had threatened to thrash 'the Chief' – the headmaster at the Institute – with her umbrella if he beat any of us! Little did she realise or ever know what fate had in store for us in Coleraine. My father, of course, who had been at the same school, said nothing and relied on us to accept what came.

Fortunately, Derek had passed the entrance examination to the school in Coleraine and was due to depart there in the following autumn. Now it was my turn to think about exams. So I had to have extra tuition as

I would have no hope of passing at my present standard. I even had to resort to doing homework, with my scruffy white friend "Mike", ever present at my feet. If it was not for his company I am sure that I would never have settled down to work.

It was a lonely winter for me after Derek, my good companion, departed for Ireland. I spent much of my time trout fishing in Tromode. Here the river was shallow enough to enable me to stalk my prey with dry fly or the upstream wet fly. I could pinpoint almost every likely spot on the river up to the Baldwin valley.

With time on my hands I would find the lies of the sea trout on their journey up the river to spawn. Returning home empty handed or with two or three nice fish did not matter to me, I was in complete harmony with nature.

I loved the wild places with only the birds and trees as company. The calls of blackbird and thrush as they tried to divert me from their nests. The swallows skimming the water to scoop fly from the rippled surface. Most of all I was enchanted by the ever-changing river with its eternal melody as it chuckled and splashed its route to the embrace of the awaiting sea.

Even now I savour the same pleasures as I walk beside a stream, observing the ephemeral ballet above the waters whilst the ever watchful trout dimples the surface gently, almost apologetically, as he sucks down any insects careless enough to rest on its lustrous face.

Many of my friends were due to move on to boarding school at the end of the summer and all but the most enduring friendships would split up. There had been some rough times with split lips and battered skulls when we clashed.

One memorable day my friend Michael and I took on all-comers who had been baiting his much quieter twin brother Peter. The previous week the three of us had carried out a solemn ceremony on the football field when we pricked our fingers and mixed our blood to become blood brothers! History does not record any victors on that day but I can recall coming out of a red fury, sitting astride Ivan Cannell and battering his head on the ground. It must have been a famous victory!

I don't even remember how I explained the damage to my mother who would have become very righteous at the thought of rough boys attacking her dear little son.

Along the lane behind our house was the Co-op bakery, which was always worth a visit on a Saturday morning. As I sidled in through the side door there was the stomach-wrenching odour of new baked bread and breakfast rolls, with brittle crusts like crab shells, that you could push your finger through.

All those scrumptious little cakes that were covered with coconut, "hundreds and thousands" and just full of cherries. I would hang around offering to carry out the most menial of tasks with the hope of some reward.

After a successful morning the bakers would send me home with tummy and pockets bulging with loot.

A short bicycle ride down the back lanes would end up at the stables where they kept some of the tram horses during the winter. The smell of horses, sweet hay and horse manure mingled together to give me an overwhelming sense of pleasure. I was overawed by the enormity of these Clydesdales and Shires with their great fluffy feet. They looked so big that I would have looked like a pimple on their backs. There they would stand in their stalls, contentedly munching away at their oats and hay, as quiet and gentle as little lambs.

"Keep out of the way as they're turnin' boy, or you'll get crushed with their great feet!" was the warning that was constantly shouted out. They were a bit bigger than Mr Marshall's riding ponies in Port Erin, so I would hastily disappear into the tack room at the back. It was full of shining hames and brasses, collars and traces and had an atmosphere of its own with the unmistakable smell of neatsfoot oil and saddle soap. The grooms spent many hours in there, keeping the harness presentable for public display

The local dairy in Spring Gardens was not far away and I could while away many hours watching the milk being prepared. The delivery lorries would arrive loaded with milk churns. All the milk would then be poured into a large tank from which it would be pasteurised by running it out over heated plates to kill off many of the bacteria and then rapidly cooled down to improve the milk's keeping qualities.

Yesterday's used milk bottles would be put into a washing machine where they would all be cleaned, scrubbed with bottle brushes, and sterilised. After a few minutes they would be trundled out in line on an endless belt, all clean and shiny, like a row of well-scrubbed schoolboys being marched into church.

On they would tinkle and rattle until they reached the filling machine when a rubber-tipped arm would descend from above and squirt the right quantity of milk into the bottle. After a couple more bangs and rattles another arm would come down to push on a cardboard cap, sealing the bottle, which then jiggled its merry way to the end of the line where it was lifted out manually and put into a milk crate, ready for delivery.

Fascinated by the progress of milk and bottles through the dairy, and overawed by the engineering that could co-ordinate the milk and sterilised bottles, I spent many hours watching and wondering which lever and gear worked the next process. It was a curiosity concerning the progress of the milk from cow to consumer that was intriguing me and probably guiding my thoughts towards farming.

Sometimes if I was at a loose end I would go off on my bike, (which had cost all of £2-10s second hand). I would cycle all over Douglas and Onchan, discovering all the byways and back roads. Out along the promenade I would pass all the men's internment camps, German,

Italian and Japanese. It was always amusing to us that when we passed the Japanese camp and it started to rain, a forest of umbrellas would appear.

My father was the medical officer for an Italian camp and used to receive Christmas cards from many of the internees following their release after the war. It did occur to us that they were probably better off being safely interned than being persecuted for their birth if they remained free.

Although many of the first internees had been brought up in the British Isles and spoke with pronounced Scots accents, others were Germans of Jewish or Aryan descent who had fled Nazi persecution. Initially, there were about 14,000 aliens in the camps throughout the island in the rush to take possible enemy agents out of circulation.

Once the authorities had considered each case individually the numbers had dropped appreciatively by January 1941.

The navy occupied Cunningham's Holiday Camp in Victoria Road and it was a source of great pride to me that, when I joined the sea scouts at 12-years-old, I had to report there for a hat as my head was too big for a boy size hat. No wonder that Bert Reid, my headmaster, had referred to me, affectionately, as Big Nut!

The Villiers Hotel was taken over by the army for training young officer cadets. They used to train in various places across the island but if we watched with binoculars from the bedroom in our house in West View we could see them carrying out hand grenade practice on the Nunnery Howe, a headland above Douglas harbour.

Of course this room had identification silhouettes of all allied and enemy planes stuck up on the wall. We knew them all off by heart and each wanted to be the one to see the first German spy plane flying over. They never did come, although we did have one raid where a plane jettisoned his bombs on the island to avoid pursuit from our fighters. The only victim that they ever located was a rather burnt frog!

I was in the house during that raid and the very brave Red Cross cycle orderly stood in the basement with his knees visibly knocking together as he did not have brother Derek to join him in being frightened.

The Sefton Hotel was taken over by the navy and re-named HMS Valkyrie. Each day squads of naval personnel used to march up to Douglas Head for training. We didn't realise that we had the first radar training station in Britain on our doorstep. More than 800 radar operators were trained in that unit.

Mum and dad entertained many of members of the forces. My mother, quite rightly, realised that that they would appreciate a bit of home cooking and the chance to meet other people. We had a number of trainee army officers visit us, which pleased my sister greatly, and regular visits by fighter pilots.

These young pilots spent a long time on duty in England and would phone us up as their 48-hour leave came up. They would fly over to Jurby airfield in the north of the island, drive down to see us and immediately go to bed for twenty-four hours.

The next morning they would be awake early, and throw us out of the nursery so that they could concentrate on playing with our electric trains until lunch time. Sunday lunch would go down with a couple of pints of beer in order that they could settle down to the serious business of a game of cricket in our sitting room with a bat and ping pong ball. We would be sent to bed early whilst they partied all evening before leaving at midnight, ready to fly back into action next day.

These were very enjoyable times when life was lived for the day, but we always felt sad when some of the pilots never returned! As children these men were our heroes and rôle models.

Chapter Five

I SPENT A LOT of my time alone, after the incident with the policeman's car. Cycling down to Tromode was always a good adventure. I would spend hours at the waterfall, watching the sea trout moving upstream. On the flat stretch up above there was a bush growing out of the wall. By carefully parting the branches I was sometimes able to see the dark silhouette of a salmon, lying tight against the wall after leaping the falls, resting before the rest of his journey upstream to spawn.

This was also the spot to collect "conkers" from the enormous horse chestnut trees in the adjacent meadow. All it required was a stout stick and a good eye to knock them down. After arriving back home, with pockets bulging, we would skewer the chestnuts, soak them in vinegar and then dry them out slowly in the oven until they were hard enough for competition.

Our pleasures were fairly simple and the school year could be divided into the "conker" season, marble season and periods when we played with tops and hoops. School was a secondary complication and approaching puberty had not intruded on our lives with serious affairs of the heart.

Sport didn't rate very highly at this stage. I found it much more intriguing to dig for pignuts on the sports field or light a fire under a wasps' nest, to smoke them out, so that we could dissect this delicate piece of architecture in nature study class. When one examines such workmanship it makes one wonder at the magic of creation and the tiny part we play in it.

At one stage we had a fad for collecting snails from the stone walls, to give to the Italian internees working on the playing field, as we heard that they ate such strange delicacies!

Further out than the waterfall was Tromode laundry, just beside the large murky pool under the bridge. This was always discoloured by the effluent from the laundry, and many times I fished there without reward.

As evening fell it would acquire an atmosphere of its own. Under the dark shadow of the bridge the air would come alive with the high-pitched squeak of bats, flitting back and forth in pursuit of moths. I used to find it eerie but compelling and fascinating just to watch their aerial ballet in almost complete silence.

Even more spine-chilling was to fish the rough water below the waterfall after dark. I would be standing alone, concentrating on my fishing when I would suddenly become aware of the wind gently rustling through the trees behind me, the moon casting dark shadows between the trees. I would have to stop fishing as every dark shadow became a threat.

I used to revel in going to the cinema with dad to see the horror films including "Cry of the Werewolf", "Dracula" and "The Black Cat".

These would become distinct possibilities the longer that I lingered in the wood, causing a rapid repetition of the Lord's Prayer and off home on my bike to reality

Sometimes I would cycle past the laundry to the millrace up above. Here, lying quietly on the bank in the evening sun I would watch the fat trout, suspended in the swiftly-flowing water, waiting for a beetle or one of the hovering flies to drop out of the overhanging trees. A quick swirl and a splash signalled the capture of yet one more delectable morsel.

From there, I could walk over the waterfalls at the head of the millstream towards the "Dubh", a dark pool at the foot of Scout's Glen, where lurked fish so large that they grew bigger with the telling. I have never landed one of these fish, but on one memorable evening I hooked a fish that irresistibly bored through the water, bending my rod double, before breaking my line on an under-water snag and leaving me shaking on the bank.

These spots were the places to test one's skill against the wily trout on a bright summer's day, or even to be rewarded with a lusty sea trout, the thoroughbred of all fishes! It was on such a beautiful day that I was dry fly fishing along the river bank in a meadow. There were some attractive little runs and eddies in the stream where there was still the ever present hope of hooking a hard-fighting brown trout, despite the brightness of the sky.

Fish caught in these conditions always give the greatest thrill as they live in a constant and variable current and, like athletes, their muscles and senses are fine tuned to a high degree.

I had already caught a couple of red speckled beauties but was constantly suffering the attentions of Alfie Kinrade's Shorthorn heifers that were grazing the pasture. These heifers had curiosity stamped over their faces and would not leave me alone. Their long, rough tongues were always ready to caress my fishing bag or leave a friendly line of slobber across my jacket. I was constantly shooing them away.

In desperation I chased them across the meadow and returned to the head of a pool where a good fish was feeding steadily. After several false casts he swirled at my fly and I made my decisive now-or-never cast. There was a scream from the reel and my rod bent double as I hooked – not a fish – but a cow that had approached too close and ended up with my fly, a beautiful Wickhams Fancy, stuck firmly in her rump.

Faced with this dilemma I sprinted towards the unfortunate animal, who strongly objected to being hooked, and headed across the field towards her companions. I put up a creditable performance and was overhauling my catch, reeling in my line when nature intervened. These gorgeous summer pastures are freckled with large numbers of soft cow pats, which are very slippery if stood on by runners in wellington boots! I fell flat on my face and my rod went merrily bouncing over the tussocks until mercifully the line broke under the strain. Not every angler can boast that he lost a 1,000 pounder!

Some days were not for angling and I would cycle on towards Kirk Braddan, returning home via Quarterbridge and Belmont Hill, to inspect the vegetables on our allotment, now occupied by Ballakermeen school!

That year, when I remained at home, was very lonely for me and I was overjoyed when everyone came back on holiday. My teacher, May Lace, must have taken compassion on me also as she invited me and Brian Kneale, later to become a successful sculptor, to her cottage at Pooilvaish once or twice.

The cottage was only a hundred yards from the sea and provided a good spot for searching rock pools or watching the Eider and Shelducks that fed around the tide's edge. I think that spot must have lots of little crabs and mussels, which are their favourite dish!

That summer was very warm, and as my sister and brothers were beginning to show an interest in tennis, so consequently we spent many days at the "Rec" tennis courts, long afternoons swimming in the sea off Broadway or just lazing on the beach. Travelling across the town so much made us very aware of the roads and back lanes in Douglas and interesting ports of call, such as Derby Road post office which had a great variety of sweets and the Bon Ton Stores, its windows packed with a fascinating mixture of hardware and household goods. There was another little grocery store tucked into a back lane off Woodburn Road that was a good stopping-off shop on the way back from school and also the site of a very sad event in later years.

Soon after qualifying as a vet some 13 years later, I was called out to this shop one winter evening, by the owners George and Daisy Kaighin, to see their aged Jack Russell Terrier, Danny, who was not well. Danny was very much loved by them and I had been involved with him as a student, since he was a puppy 13 years before.

George and Daisy were about 70 years of age and made a small but diminishing income as a neighbourhood store. I arrived at the shop and was shown into the back room by Daisy to find George listening to the radio. Daisy was quite small, round and jolly with steel rimmed spectacles whereas George was equally small but thin, with a weather-beaten face after many years spent as a council roadman.

As I entered the tiny room, I could have cut the air with a knife. The heat from the blazing fire combined with the fumes of the plug tobacco from George's pipe were enough to kill a donkey.

Danny was in his box by the fireside, well wrapped up in a blanket. "What's the trouble with our little friend tonight?", I said in a concerned manner.

"It's like this Mr Vet ," said George. "You know how our Danny has been troubled with his walking over the past two years. Well, he's been getting slower of late and had a cough as if he had something jammed in his throat.

"Four days ago he went off his food and didn't want to go for a walk. Next day he lay in bed and lapped a little broth, so we wrapped him up comfortably. Since then he's not wanted to eat or go for a walk and we didn't want to call out a busy man like yourself over the weekend."

As I knelt down beside Danny he didn't make his usual move to greet me. I unfolded the covering blanket only to confirm my worst fears. Danny had been dead for possibly two days and his bloated body was already decomposing in the hot room. I was at a loss for words and went through the motions of examining him whilst I thought deeply.

I turned round to Daisy and George who were clasping hands on the sofa. "I'm afraid old friends that Danny has just slipped away gently and quietly." At his age it would have been well-nigh impossible to help him enjoy life as I suspect that he had developed heart problems and could never have been active again.

Daisy went over and, sobbing quietly, stroked Danny's grizzled head whilst George blew his nose hard and set to restoking his pipe. Daisy interrupted the silence, "Thank you for coming mister, we knew that this day was not far off. I don't know what George will do as he used to take Danny to the Woodburn Hotel for a pint each evening. We have a little plot at the back where George will dig a hole in the morning."

I went home with a heavy heart as I found myself getting emotionally involved with the Kaighin's problems. Had one of them realised that Danny had died beforehand and made no mention for fear of upsetting the other? After all he was the only child of this devoted couple and would leave a big gap in their lives.

Chapter Six

RAINY DAYS ARE always a problem for active youngsters and we were no exception. Fortunately, we had been brought up to enjoy each other's company and could spend hours playing card games or darts in our basement nursery. Mum was quite clever at diverting us when she was cooking. We would be drafted into the kitchen to help make cakes, drop scones or "fadge", the Irish potato bread.

All of my mother's spare time was spent in the kitchen preparing food for her hungry brood. She was determined that her beloved husband would be well looked after, as he was working such long hours. When harvest time arrived she would order in large quantities of fruit. Row upon row of Kilner jars would take over the kitchen table to await their fate.

We would all be enlisted into the production line to assist, chop up fruit and fill the bottles. The bottles of fruit were then stood in a large pan of water and were brought to the boil. They were then topped with rubber seals and a glass top, held on firmly by a screw cap. Dad had bottled fruit for breakfast every day during the war, and any family rejoicing was always celebrated by opening an extra Kilner jar.

When the war commenced mum also put down a bread crock full of eggs in Isinglass, which lasted for many months. Early on we had had a ham preserved and hung in the attic, although rationing in the island was never as severe as that on the mainland. It was always possible to obtain a few extras in the way of meat and dairy products.

This was a result of the island's farm production being geared to the holiday industry, which was now non-existent. Consequently there was often a surplus of food in the island and most people could exceed their ration. It was always a bone of contention that many of the internees who were comparatively wealthy, could live better than the locals!

We had gone out of the house after one particularly stormy night to discover that our lilac tree had been split from top to bottom by lightning. This occurrence stimulated our curiosity about the power of nature.

I was rather frightened at the thought of the near miss that might have struck the house as I had just been reading about "fireballs" resulting from electric storms. I think that I had a word with God about it, but He didn't seem to be much help at the time.

Following this incident we all became born-again scientists and wanted to know how and why things worked. When Christmas came Ted had a stationary steam engine where he heated up the boiler and steam hissed out, causing wheels to go round and pistons and pulleys to start working.

Derek had a chemistry set with all sorts of interesting experiments which one could carry out. As a result of his experimentation we spent months moving rugs around the bedroom floor to cover up acid burns through the carpet where there had been small errors.

Cecile had music books as she was in love for the first time with an officer cadet, and we had to listen to soppy tunes such as "Among my Souvenirs" and "The Badge from your Coat" being played incessantly on the piano! As a younger brother I just could not understand this dramatic change from a tomboy sister to a young teenager. Girls did seem to become very silly, sometimes!

I was considered as being too dangerous to handle a chemistry set. It didn't worry me much as I had discovered reading. "The Outline of Nature," "Romance of the Nation", and "Wonders of the World" were all avidly digested. Nobody could believe that I was becoming interested in knowledge, but I was also entering that dangerous age of enquiry and experimentation!

I was intrigued by the theory of gravity and the earth's rotation. Did this account for rain coming down at an angle? But sometimes it came down straight and why did milk fall straight from a milk jug? The problems were immeasurable for a budding scientist! I hung a weighted piece of string out of my third storey bedroom window but as it hung vertically it was of no help to my research. In theory the cord should have hung at an angle due to the world's rotation.

After some discussion with my brothers I developed a new theory. We went up to the fourth storey landing from which we could peer over the edge and see the distant floor, four storeys down, through a narrow gap separating the descending banisters. The floor at the bottom was just outside the room where the patients waited to see my father.

The cord and pendulum hung vertically like a plumb line for four storeys. So, the weight was too heavy! Then we decided to try feathers which we extracted from mum's pillows. They were too light and drifted away with every draught.

Then came the ultimate idea. A good blob of spit proved to be just the correct weight and could be watched as it plunged slowly and inexorably downwards until eventually it hit the ground with a rather satisfying sound. This was so exciting and was so endlessly repeatable that I almost became dehydrated. How many times out of a hundred did spittle deviate away from the vertical?

This experiment went on for several days until a patient suggested to my father that the roof must be leaking. My father was a quiet man normally. Consequently, when he raised his voice and fixed me with his steel blue eyes (which he inherited from my grandmother!), I quaked with fear. Physical punishment was not required.

This was the first time that I had been frightened by him since the day that I mixed pepper into the sugar bowl during the first week of food rationing. I was really concerned that adults found it difficult to enjoy a joke! It took me several hours to wash, clean and polish the banisters, although I was a bit put out to find that, in addition, my bike had been confiscated for a week.

Like all budding scientists I was fascinated by the theories of the trajectory and aim as applied to bullets and arrows. I never could get an arrow to fly straight. A further development was to use a hollow brass stair rod as a means of hunting, using sago or dried peas. My friends soon got fed up with being hit by dried peas as I crouched in my hide in the privet hedge. I did frighten a few low flying seagulls using sago bullets.

I was quietly sitting in my bedroom one evening reading a book when I was constantly interrupted by caterwauling outside. Looking out of my third storey window I could see our cat 'Spats' confronting an enormous tabby cat with a turnip head, which denoted a full tom cat.

Fearing for his safety I shouted at them, but they were too involved challenging one another. I picked up a glass marble in the hope of scaring the intruder. As fate would have it at that moment, the invader moved three feet backwards and Spats moved forwards only for the marble to hit him on the head. Spats gave a squawk, staggered sideways and the invader fled, suspecting that this was a devious manoeuvre to outwit him.

Chapter Seven

EARLY IN MAY mum and I set out on the 'Mona's Isle', one of the few ships left in service from the island, and eventually arrived in Fleetwood after a rather rough journey that left us feeling a bit weak – although I did not spot any U-boats! This was the first part of my journey to take the entrance examinations at Coleraine 'Inst',

From Fleetwood we went by train to Preston where we had a six-hour wait for our connection to Heysham. Preston station, during the war, was a cold and miserable place to be so we went into town, found a cinema and watched a film about people kissing, crying and waving good-bye at a railway station as the man went off to war in navy uniform.

As a young man of the world I found such behaviour very strange indeed. We then had a meal in a rather dingy and depressed-looking hotel with several other diners picking at spam and soggy-looking cabbage in a rather desultory manner. The waitresses looked old and tired, rather like the hotel itself! Mum explained that this was caused by the wartime food shortage, and the tired waitresses were probably also working at night as fire watchers or air raid wardens.

War took on a different meaning for me and I realised just how lucky we were in the island, where rationing was not nearly as severe. I had asked who had given us the sheepskin rugs at home only to be told that several sheep had died. There must have been a very flourishing market in sheepskins in the island at that time as mutton was not an uncommon addition to the menu.

Tom Brew, the butcher along the terrace, was held in great esteem during those years and managed to look after his customers very well. It was he who taught me how to make sausages using a hand mincing machine and a long length of sausage skin.

After our meal we took a taxi back to the station and arrived shortly before our train was due. Every railway station seemed to be packed with soldiers, sailors and airmen heading in different directions, with a fair sprinkling of young women looking very smart in their uniforms. Civilians were almost in a minority and the crush on the trains was exhausting.

Our train to Heysham pulled in and as quickly as the carriages emptied they seemed to fill up again. Every carriage and all the corridors were full of people standing and holding on tightly as the train lurched from side to side.

The era of politeness and courtesy to ladies was still with us and, in spite of the fatigue and stress on the men's faces, women were offered seats, particularly if they were young, pretty and in uniform. I stood in the corridor with the men whilst mum found a seat in a nearby carriage.

We arrived in Heysham soon after eight p.m. and joined the customs queue for the overnight boat for Belfast. I had never been through customs before and was fascinated watching the men go through people's baggage, stamping the passes and waving them through to the ticket office. I did notice that there were a couple of ladies at the end also looking through bags. They had kind faces, not nearly as stern as the men.

Once on board we were shown our cabin and before settling down for the night we went for a walk on deck. There were uniforms everywhere. People leaning over the rail taking a last look at shore, chatted up pretty A.T.S. girls or had a last smoke before turning in. Down below in the steerage there was a group of sailors singing "Roll out the Barrel" to the strains of a mouth organ with a large rascally-looking, black-bearded sailor waving his arms in the air, conducting the orchestra, whilst in the background there was a lot of laughter and shouting from the direction of the bar.

Noticing as we looked over the rail to the stern part of the boat that many people were already stretched out on the wooden seats below preparing to sleep. "Why aren't they in cabins mum?"

"They are the poor people travelling steerage who cannot afford a cabin," she replied. This comment made me think deeply on the divisions amongst people. I already had this partly-formed impression in my mind that she was a snob, rather involved in her own importance. Why did she always insist on being addressed as Mrs Dr Stuart? I didn't know anyone else like that!

We were both fairly tired and it didn't take long for me to fall asleep, despite the strangeness of the rolling and banging which takes place in a ship at sea. When we awoke next morning the ship was already unloading in the docks in Belfast. After a light breakfast we hired a taxi to take us along Corporation Street to the railway station.

As we settled in the train I noticed that quite a few of the sailors in the carriage had been on the boat at Heysham the previous night, including "Blackbeard", looking very much more subdued. I wondered whether he had been a pirate in peace time!

The train seemed to take a long time to reach Coleraine as it stopped at so many stations, one of which struck me as a comical name – Culleybackey Junction.

When we alighted at Coleraine it was nice to see "Adden", as we called Aunt Ivy, at the station to meet us. She gave me a big hug as she had not seen me for several years. We loaded our cases into the car and in five minutes we arrived at Hanover Place, where my grandparents lived.

I had always been very fond of my grandparents. "Dando", my grandfather, loved children, and had a very mischievous sense of humour, so teased us unmercifully. I was always warned when visiting gran that I should not mention beer or whiskey in her presence, nor talk about playing cards for money as she was very strictly religious in her views. It did cramp my style a bit even though I was her blue-eyed boy, so much so that she would have liked to see me become a Presbyterian minister like Great Uncle John in Derry. I never did feel that I had a true calling as a man of the cloth – better to be a missionary and lie in the sun!

It was always fun to visit gran when she spent a few days in bed. I felt that this was the normal thing for very old ladies to do periodically. Her room always had an "Old Lady" smell to it, mixed with the odour of lavender and mothballs. On the wall was a gadget with a whistle attached to a speaking tube in order that she could call to the kitchen from her bedroom to issue instructions to the servants.

Whenever she left the house, Derek and I would take over the bedroom and kitchen to re-enact the great naval battles and give orders to the engine room such as "Dive, dive, dive!" or " Hard a'port Mr Jones, enemy submarines on port bow. Prepare to attack". This is how we won the battle of the Irish Sea!

Orders could also be sent to the engine room by rushing between bedrooms, and pulling the bell handles, which rang like a carillon on the bell board in the kitchen. We had nominated Lizzie, the ancient cook, as the Chief Stoker, but even her tolerance ran out in the end when we would be chased out of her kitchen.

Next morning Adden drove me up to the Coleraine Academical Institution. The name itself was overwhelming and smattered of serious academic pursuits with a touch of Tom Brown's schooldays. As the car turned into the drive I could see this large imposing yellow building that might have been part of a Georgian mansion with a wide flight of steps running down to the gravelled driveway. On either side the school wings flared out in an Lshape which immediately dispelled the illusion but inferred an impression of permanence. Grassy slopes flanked the school on three sides whilst a gravelled path continued down from the steps, through a monumental archway to the wide expanse of the cricket field.

I remember little of the examination as I was overwhelmed by the grandeur of the place. I was told that exam results would be out in July. Our subsequent tour through the dormitories and boarding facilities showed me that they were quite sparse and I wished that I was safe in my bedroom at home listening to the familiar and lonely moaning of the foghorn on Douglas Head.

I was very pleased to return to my grandparents' house where we stayed for a few more days. I used to spend hours playing Bezique with my grandfather and every time that I beat him he threatened to send me away to a sweet factory with a muzzle on or give me an attack of that dreaded disease, "Fearbellurgan".

One of my lasting impressions of Ulster, at that time, was the religious divide. I had been brought up with a great sense of fairness and acceptance of other people in society (unless they had snotty noses!). I was completely bewildered by the dominance of Orangeism and the denigration of the Catholics. Apart from one very tolerant Catholic boy, Frank Trufelli, all the pupils were Protestant. I did not come into contact with any Catholics amongst my peers until I went to Queen's University.

When several of my friends told me that they could know a Catholic just by looking at him I was even more confused as I did not possess this magic insight. My sister later told me that it was because the Catholics were poorer and less well dressed as they always received the menial jobs. I was told not to enter Killowen, the poorer part of Coleraine, lest I might be set upon.

On a weekend pass from school I would stay at my grandparents in Hanover Place and I mentioned my worries to my Aunt Adden.

"Yes!" She said. "Jimmy (her boyfriend) and I have had to live with this problem but it is changing and people are becoming more tolerant. Your grandfather's parents were brought up in this very bigoted atmosphere. When he went into business on his own he found that half of his customers were Catholic.

Being a very even handed man he was increasingly concerned about the situation. To salve his conscience and treat his clients equally he left the Black Preceptor, and the Orange order and never attended the Presbyterian Church again." To carry out such an act in 1926, so soon after the troubles, was indeed a very brave thing to do, but it seemed to pay dividends for his business.

It was he who told me about the corrupt practice of 'gerrymandering', whereby a wealthier man, i.e. protestant, could buy a garden hut in each province, which automatically gave him a vote in that area to keep the Catholics in a minority!

As a little boy I would lie in bed at Hannover listening to the incessant beating of the Orangemen's Lambeg drums across the river in Killowen. This noise would continue for hours. As one of my friends said, it was a way of proving their allegiance to the Crown. I found it most intimidating that people were so misguided and unintelligent.

My grandmother, a Carson from Ballymena, was of a different mould. A stalwart Presbyterian, she repeatedly signed the pledge during her lifetime to confirm solidarity with the church. She did upset my aunt by throwing away a perfectly good Christmas cake away lest it might contain alcohol. Little did she realise that she had been bequeathed a street in Ballymena, which contained nine pubs!

She once confided to me that Catholics were really quite nice people. 'It's a pity that they are all thieves and liars!' Thank goodness that those days are past. I listened to her playing hymns on the piano at ninety-years old and singing in a high-pitched falsetto. Despite our differences in age and belief, I held her in great esteem for her wisdom.

One day her nurse, Renee, a lovely large lady from Cork, asked gran when she was dressing her where she had put her large brassy brooch, only to be corrected, firmly, that it was an '18 carat gold love knot' – whoops!

In contrast, Dando, then 84, called her across the landing to his room 'Nurse, nurse – come quickly'. Renee rushed across, expecting to find him in extremis. 'Mr Stuart! What is it at all?'

He was sitting up in bed with eyes twinkling. 'Ach ! Jump into bed with me!' She never did tell me the rest, but next morning he was found dead in bed. Quel joie!

The 'Picture Post' was a popular weekly photographic magazine of the time. Whenever Adden bought a copy gran would make 'tutting' sounds and suggest that it was hidden away, lest it might influence my morality. All parties were eventually satisfied as my aunt would show me where she had hidden it after gran had gone to bed.

It was not long after our Coleraine visit that the family arrived home on summer holidays. I had so many questions to ask my brothers about the school that in the end they suspected that I was a little bit worried about this next big adventure. I did, however, feel quite grown up as my voice had just broken, having gone through that embarrassing squeaky stage. Like all brothers they would put me down if I was too cocky by speaking in French, their newly acquired tongue.

In July I learnt that I had been accepted at 'Inst.' despite my lack of academic prowess in the exams. My marks in the maths paper were 50 out of 500, which was not quite what my mother had expected.

However, I resolved to be philosophical about the situation as this gave me an opportunity for great improvement. I realised that I could not compete with my elder siblings as they were fairly bright. For years I had suffered the comments of my elders when they said, "I should hope that you are as clever as your brother". This made me so cross that I decided that I would never be a swot!

We went through about six weeks of exceptionally hot weather that summer with simmering heat day after day. There was a haze over the countryside and the road surface rippled with the heat and melting tar. Even fishing lost its allure during the day and I would have to wait for the evening rise. In the bright sunshine I would lie on the river bank, basking in the heat like a lizard.

Looking upwards, into the pale blue mantle of the heavens, I would watch the skylark's tenuous ascent until it was almost out of sight although the sound of its haunting and tremulous song never faded.

Perhaps that is why the fish were still, captured by the magic of this tiny bird chanting forth its paeon of joy! The drowsy humming of insects was like so many stringed instruments supporting this diva of the sky.

The world was at peace on such days with only the odd Hurricane or Spitfire almost lazily joining in a mock dogfight high in the heavens above me. Yet these glorious days were a continuation of the Battle of Britain days, when our airmen were fighting along the south coast for air supremacy and freedom.

Our weekend visitors and heroes, Drummond Wilson and Arthur Cross were amongst them! Please God, let them come back! I had felt very strongly since looking out of my bedroom window one night in May and seeing a glow in the sky across Douglas bay.

Later, I had been told that it was Liverpool, ninety miles away, burning after the German bombers had blasted the heart out of Bootle and the docks. To make it worse they hit Bryant and Mays match factory which was like a giant firework.

Life was much easier for my father and in this sunny spell he would arrange a consultancy in Ramsey on a Sunday. In this manner, his business petrol would enable us all to go for a picnic on the banks of the Sulby river at Milntown, where he would fish until the evening rise and I would plod along behind as his ghillie.

We took a schoolteacher friend of my mother on one of these picnics with the express purpose of collecting as many blackberries as possible for jam-making. This particular lady was a rather large, middle-aged schoolteacher, who was very excited over the prospect of a day out. I suppose one could say that she was graceful when she moved, like a galleon in full sail. Dad and I went fishing nearby and left our friend Georgie and my mother to collect blackberries.

After ten minutes the evening calm was shattered by the most unladylike screams. I ran up the field towards them and found my mother clinging to the field gate in paroxysms of laughter. Georgie had climbed over the gate, on the principle that the grass over the fence is always greener. Sure enough, there were blackberries aplenty and she was soon filling her containers. Unfortunately, the farmer, Juan Callow, had omitted to warn them that his pet Suffolk ram was loose in the field.

Sam the ram had wandered over to Georgie in his normal friendly manner, with memories of bottles of milk, when he was a hand-fed lamb. When nothing was forthcoming, like a spoilt child, he walked up behind and butted her bottom as a reminder. Those valuable blackberries were scattered far and wide as Georgie's hands went to protect her bottom. Each time she shrieked he gave her another butt with his extremely hard head for good measure. By the time I had restrained Sam, Georgie was a deep scarlet under her liberal makeup and in a state bordering on hysteria. Suffice to say that like all good stories, the tale grew more interesting with each telling.

Chapter Eight

AT HOME ALL was busy as my mother prepared for the last of her brood to leave the nest. There were great goings on as she and my sister collected all my school kit together. Two grey suits (short trousers), gabardine raincoat, school blazer from Tweedy Acheson's resplendent with red, white and blue stripes, and a large school cap with badge, which I always felt resembled a Guinness label.

Grey shirts, ties, pyjamas and travelling rug; socks and two pairs of black shoes had to be accounted for as well as underwear. All these had to have special name labels stitched onto them. That was the part that mum disliked!

In addition, mum insisted that I took body belts and liberty bodices that had been compulsory garb since I had had TB. I never did tell her that they remained in the bottom of my locker – too cissy! All our school trunks were sent off a week early in order that they arrived at school before us.

Before heading for school I casually asked mum what job her dad had done. After some hesitation she said that he was in the ironmongery business (n.b. not trade). I took this all in and later asked my Welsh aunt what he did. She immediately said that he served behind the counter in a hardware shop. The truth was out! My mother was ashamed of her humble beginnings and developed her snobbery after marrying a doctor.

A bright sun greeted the morning of 3rd of September 1943, which made my departure from the land of my birth even more poignant. All of those long cycle rides and adventures around Douglas were put on hold!

Rather dilapidated, the "Mona's Isle" reflected the lack of care as she was one of the remaining steam packet ships left in service. Already we had lost the 'Mona's Queen' at Dunkirk and the other members of the fleet were too busy to warrant a refit. A steady line of passengers filed up the gangway, encumbered with suitcases and kit bags.

After lingering too long at the ticket barrier, talking the usual trivialities, we each gave Mum and Dad a hug before we left. The other three were given last minute instructions to take care of me and make sure that I kept out of trouble. A vain hope! Sometimes, I wondered why I should always be the one to end up in predicaments!

I was trying to be particularly brave, as I walked up the gangplank, with a lump in my throat and a deep anguish in my very soul as I stepped off the quay side. We had a cabin reserved for ourselves and the baggage although I suspected that they all thought that I would lie there feeling seasick.

As the ship cast off and slowly slipped out of the harbour, I stood at the rail, eyes dimmed with tears and rather afraid of what might be in store for me. The sea, shimmering blue in the autumn sun, was as calm as a mill pond.

The spring tide all but covered the Conister Rock, leaving the Tower of Refuge in splendid isolation, with the impressive backdrop of Douglas Bay, curving across from the Fort Anne Hotel, which dominated the harbour, to Port Jack in the distance.

I stayed at the stern rail for a long time, saying my farewells as the island slipped away behind until it became but a purple cloud on the horizon. Even the herring gulls, scavenging in the wake, gradually dropped away. Jane came and joined me for a few minutes and said happily, "Come on. The buffet's open soon. How about a cup of tea and sausage rolls in the lounge?"

We fought our way along the deck, crowded with troops and sailors en-route to another posting. Piles of kit bags and a couple of army lorries blocked the way as we pushed past the crowded bar into the lounge.

Here we had to queue at the buffet, behind several wrens, returning to their units from the signals training school in Douglas. As we waited, Ted and Derek went off to bag a table and spread themselves across the seats.

When we eventually sat down to have our snack, Ted explained to me, "On these journeys you have to learn to look after yourself. We rushed off to grab this table, otherwise you would have had to stand. When you are in a group you can cut a lot of corners if you work as a team."

The journey was remarkably smooth and swift and by early afternoon we had berthed in Fleetwood. Collecting our baggage we rushed for the train, clambered on board, and set off for Preston. Once again the train was full of troops, but by group power we managed to find two seats in a compartment. This did not last long as two middle-aged mums, loaded with shopping, staggered along the corridor so we offered them our seats.

As we drew into Preston station, I remembered how shocked I had been on my previous journey to see what seemed to be street after street of little grimy red brick houses standing back to back. They all had small back yards with washing hanging out and doors that opened into tiny back lanes.

A thick pall of smoke hung over the whole town filtering away the sunlight. When I thought back to Glen Mooar and Port Erin with the green fields, sea and clear air I realised just how lucky I was to have been born on the island. I still have this strong feeling of belonging to my Celtic roots.

A quirk of fate and I might have been brought up in Preston in 1930! Years later, in philosophical mood, I wondered that if the world had gone through another quarter rotation, whether I might have been born to someone in Mongolia!

As we drew into the station, Ted, always the organiser, said: "Come on! All cases into the left luggage office and with a bit of luck we can get in a meal and two films before our train leaves for Heysham" – much better than sitting around in a miserable station for six hours. We managed to see a full-length cartoon, have a meal and then watch another film about the navy chasing the German pocket battleships.

We had found a rather worn out looking café for our meal. The front windows were covered with a criss-cross of sticky tape to protect against bomb blast. The inside was dark and smelt of stale chip fat. The tables were covered with greasy worn oilcloth and the unwashed floor covered with dirty linoleum.

It was a case of any port in a storm, so we settled for some bully beef, soggy potatoes and depressed-looking cabbage. The meal was finished off with a plate of stale grey bread covered with a slick of margarine, and a cup of tea to wash it all down.

Hurrying back to the station, we just had time to bail out our luggage before the train for Heysham arrived. The station was a sea of uniforms with many weary travellers sound asleep on benches or on the ground, heads resting on their kit bags. We were caught up in the rush onto the train but this time only managed to reach the corridor where we had to sit on our cases for the remainder of the journey.

On arrival at Heysham we were faced with a long queue, waiting for the customs and emigration office to open its doors at 9 p.m. Ted turned round to Derek and me, in a conspiratorial manner. "We have nearly an hour before the customs office opens. If we are near the front we can get past the customs men to the lady at the far end. Noel, you're the smallest and will get most sympathy so you lead the way."

Slowly and casually we moved our cases forward, foot by foot. Shuffling and chatting amongst ourselves, we progressed almost imperceptibly until the doors opened and we were in the first ten in the queue. Leaving those in front of us to deal with the customs men we ran straight towards the rather maternal and sympathetic customs lady and plonked our cases in front of her.

No doubt she had seen this ploy re-enacted many times before, but she went through the motions of examining our cases very carefully, overlooking the well-wrapped cake in each case and the bars of chocolate hidden in the rolled up socks. Maybe she had a gang of scruffy kids at home as well! For me, this was the first of many trips through customs and it never lost the excitement of trying to queue jump and the game of 'let's pretend' with the customs lady!

Arriving in Belfast next morning to hear the calls of the dockers with their unmistakable Northern Irish accents was a new experience. I enjoy arriving at a new port to be greeted by different dialects but the Ulster dialect has always left me with a warm feeling, reminiscent of kindness and good cooking. A brief check at immigration of our residence permits and we struggled onto the quayside with our cases.

We were fortunate to be greeted by Jimmy Dunwoodie, my aunt's fiancé, who was a member of the Royal Ulster Constabulary. Jimmy was a big, bluff, fair-haired man with a pink and genial face. A very competent sportsman, he played rugby and golf for the RUC and was always happy in the company of young people. Under Jimmy's guidance we were taken to the Xcel Cafe in Haymarket for breakfast.

Everyone seemed to know Jimmy and he was greeted as a long lost friend when he ordered breakfast for us all. This meal was the answer to a growing boy's dreams and typical of the breakfasts which I came to expect in Ireland. After a starter consisting of a large plate of porridge, came the fried breakfast – a plate with two fried eggs, sausages, a couple of large rashers of bacon, tomato and a few pieces of fried soda farls and fadge (potato bread).

Feeling pretty good this time we were loaded onto a tram in Corporation Street that took us to the railway station and from thence to Coleraine where we arrived in the early afternoon.

Adden met us at the station and took Cecile (or Jane as she was later known) off to Coleraine High School. We took a taxi to Inst.

When we arrived at the school it was a bustle of activity. The driveway outside the schoolhouse was a kaleidoscope of red, white and blue striped blazers. Boys standing outside with their families as their bags were unloaded, others regaling one another with tales of the summer's exploits. Through this mêlée, the dominant figures of gowned masters strode, like huntsmen in a kennel, marshalling the boys and directing them to their new dormitories. At the top of the steps in a navy dress stood the matron Miss Johnson talking to a stockily-built, be-gowned master who, I was to learn later, was Major White, the headmaster.

"The Chief", formally Major William White, DSO and bar, was my headmaster in Ulster. With a ruddy complexion, wire frame spectacles and a thinning hairline, "The Chief", as he was respectfully termed, was an imposing figure with a dignity and personality to match. Regarded with awe by pupils and staff alike, he possessed an aura of command that kept us all on our toes. He always appeared in a grey suit with sparkling military shoes and many a pupil was withered by a glance from his blue eyes behind steel rimmed glasses peering from beneath beetling eyebrows, until they noticed the chuckle lines twitching at the corner of his eyes.

Apart from his daring exploits on the battlefield, he was held up as a rôle model as he had once played goalkeeper for Glasgow Rangers. That was before he crossed the Irish sea and became converted to the oval ball.

Rumours about his discipline grew into schoolboy legend, concerning the cat-o-nine-tails which he held in his cupboard that was kept freshly polished for miscreants. In the brief period when he taught me, I had an excellent opportunity to study him during the time that I should have been soaking up maths. I was fascinated by the four curly hairs which sprouted out from his rosy cheeks and the mini-moustaches curling around the edges of his nostrils.

I had been seated in the front row in order that I might be observed closely. He spoke in short explosive sentences in his broad Scots accent. Each word was accompanied by a volley of spittle projected across the front two rows of desks. I received the full impact of his aerosol effect. In the front row I could listen attentively whilst surreptitiously circling each drop of liquid that landed on my exercise book. Towards the end of one lesson he peered down at my exercise book – "What are all those little circles, Noel? (He knew all our Christian names). Is this a game of noughts and crosses?"

Terrified at being subject to his scrutiny I stammered, "No sir! I was subconsciously drawing little circles in my maths book to try and make a perfect nought" I couldn't really admit that I had been encircling each little drop of spit as it landed on my book.

"Well in that case Noel, you can stay in detention after school and write out a hundred times 'I must pay more attention during mathematics lessons' and another ten lines of perfect noughts". I was terrified at being noticed by "The Chief." It brought me one step nearer to the cat-o-nine-tails.

I received a very rapid response shortly afterwards, in the chemistry laboratory, when I connected the water tap to the gas jet and turned both taps on. Our respected headmaster was unfortunately teaching physics in the laboratory underneath and did not appreciate jets of water coming out of the bunsen burners. He suddenly appeared at the door with a face like thunder and I narrowly escaped a beating. 'C'est la vie'

One of our great joys was to see him make an error, no matter how slight, in order that we knew that he had human failings. He always got terribly involved as a spectator at rugby matches. Whilst watching a crucial cup match, our wing three quarter, "Tommy", streaked up the touch line towards a certain score, on which the game hung, only to be foully tripped by an opponent.

In the ensuing silence, the Chief was heard to roar out "Kick his arse, Tommy. Kick his arse!"

'The Chief' was there to greet any concerned parents and use his undoubted charm to assure them that the newcomers would be looked after well and made to feel at home. At this stage he would beam at Miss Johnson who would take the parents and child up to their dormitory, show them their bed and locker, and leave them to settle in whilst she went off to meet the next bright-eyed little chap. My brothers handed me over to Miss Johnson's care whilst they went off to find their own dormitories.

Struggling up the stairs after Miss Johnson with my case, gabardine raincoat and gas mask, I turned off right at the top of the stairs into the "South" dormitory where many of the new boys slept. Right across the landing was "Middle" dorm, where Derek slept, and beyond that the "North" dorm, which the sixth form, including Ted and many prefects, occupied.

When I entered "South" there were only a few other boys installed; Billy McVicker in the next bed, Don Taylor, Basil McCrea and down at the end, Robbie Patterson. Most of them were younger than I was, although I realised later that it would not have been good policy to put me in the same dorm as my brother -better to let me fight my own battles!

As mine was the end bed, I slept beside my clothes locker which was quite handy for late night feasts, although it did have the disadvantage of being nearest to the matron's quarters and the boarding staff bathroom. This meant that I had to stand at the door into Miss Johnson's quarters to act as guard whenever anything illicit was going on!

Just before tea time Sergeant "Bummer" Boyce arrived in our dormitory and introduced himself. A slightly built man of about 60 years of age, with grey hair and a bushy grey moustache, he worked on the army theory that if you frightened the boys a bit to start with he would get instant obedience later on. He was caretaker and general factotum in the school and one of his main duties was to get all the boys moving in the mornings.

He glared at us and said, "Right, youse boys. You are the first to get up in the morning to go down to the ablutions, where I shall make sure that you wash all over, particularly your hands and ears! Then you will jump into the plunge bath and walk or swim a length.

"It may seem a bit cold in the winter when it's freezing outside, particularly when you have to break the ice. Don't forget you are lucky that we don't make you roll in the snow. I shall ring the bell every morning at a quarter to seven and if I find any of you still in bed five minutes later, I shall pull off your blankets and give you the 'Red Hand of Ulster' across your bottom. Now follow me down to the dining hall for tea!"

Duly chastened we followed him down two storeys to the dining hall that was in the basement. The room itself was well lit as it had quite a few large windows. Three rows of tables stretched the length of the room. One row, next to the boarding staff table, was reserved for the senior boys. The other two were available for the rest of us. Each table had about three large copper urns of tea and several jugs of milk available.

Plates of white bread were placed along the tables and a few plates of little cupcakes from which you might see one or two currants shyly peeping through the surface. We were permitted to bring our own pots of jam or golden syrup to supplement our jam and sugar rations. It was often possible to buy jam off the ration from a wee grocery shop which served Killowen, the poorer part of town where the local people could not afford to buy their full rations. Periodically, the diet would be varied with scones or wholemeal bread made in the kitchens.

After tea we had to unpack all our cases and also the trunks that had suddenly appeared. As we unpacked, the laundry maids would take all our linen and towels, each one with the name tag sewn on for storage and make up our beds before vanishing towards the laundry room. Under the watchful eye of Miss Johnson we were shown how to pack our clothes tidily into the lockers, putting our tuck boxes, shoes and cleaning gear at the bottom.

'Lights out' was at 9 p.m., and as we changed into pyjamas we were very aware that we had never undressed in public before. As we were all starting puberty there was a great consciousness of our own bodies and also a curiosity about other boys. We were embarrassed about our developing sexuality and turned away whilst stealing furtive glimpses at our neighbours to make sure that they were made the same. One poor little guy was very under developed and had quite a bit of teasing until his testicles and voice both dropped several months later.

These conditions of awareness can result in experimentation and homosexuality in cloistered situations. Fortunately, it was virtually non-existent at Inst., possibly due to the open plan of the dormitories and the tradition for the seniors to meet their girl friends in the town at weekends or to sneak out furtively at night.

As soon as the lights went out the darkness was full of the rich Ulster dialect as each boy tried to find common acquaintances on which to base a relationship. Uncharacteristically I kept silent, just listening to the voices floating through the night and revelling in their accents. It was an ephemeral, almost out-of-body feeling of detachment as I lay and took no part in the proceedings.

I can clearly recall a long discussion between two farmer's sons on the subject of "whitrets" or weasels. Part of the folklore of whitrets was that you should never corner them if you were alone. Several stories told of such happenings when the cornered whitret put his tail in his mouth and whistled. This brought dozens of others on the scene who would attack the tormentor and drive him off. My interest was so great that gradually the voices grew fewer and fainter as I listened intently and slipped unknowingly into sleep.

The first few weeks at the school settled any problems of home sickness as the ten members of the South dorm got to know one another and form bonds of friendship. Having got over the initial week when there were a few tears we really began to enjoy the life. We learned the rules that had to be obeyed and boundaries which must not be overstepped and were quite happy with the situation.

For a couple of boys it had all been too much and they ran away, but those remaining formed a group and we used to lie in bed until all hours at night, talking and plotting various escapades. I was luckier than most, having two brothers at the school, although I was threatened with retribution a couple of times by those who had been bullied by my eldest brother.

Clang! Clang! The Angelus was sounding! I struggled out of a dreamy sleep and realised that it was the sergeant ringing the bell next morning and almost immediately he burst into the room, switched on the lights, shouting, "Come on ye boys. The last one out of bed gets the Red Hand."

Simultaneously, 10 pairs of feet hit the floor and staggered, confused and drugged with sleep towards their dressing gowns and wash bags.

"Right ye boys, follow me. If you don't get a move on you'll be late and miss your breakfast," continued the sergeant in his best regimental manner.

Like the pied piper, he led us down to the basement, past the dining hall and along the corridor to the changing room. There was no self-consciousness about our shivering bodies as he chivvied us into the plunge room. The plunge room contained a pool full of water that resembled thick coffee. I found out later that this was "peat," suspended in the water as the streams ran through the peat bogs. Even our drinking water, which was very palatable, was often stained brown.

Around the edge of the pool was a row of nearly twenty washbasins so we all stood in a line, naked as the day we were born, scrubbing ourselves and brushing teeth under the watchful eye of Sergeant Boyce. "Come on you boys, the next batch are here. Get into the plunge and either swim or walk a length if you want any breakfast".

Even in September the plunge was cold although we soon became hardened to it. One of the problems with the dark waters of the plunge was that we could not see any dead rats until we stood on them. After plunge time there was normally a stampede into the changing rooms to dry off quickly, warm up and rush back to the dormitory.

We would all come in for a bath after playing rugger and many of us went in for a swim in the plunge before drying off. The plunge was only about three feet in depth and there was always the challenge of diving in and attempting to swim two lengths under water. It had to be a very shallow dive to avoid hitting the bottom although one enthusiast tried a no-arms dive and was carried off to the sickbay with concussion.

One of the subtle means of bullying was for a group of senior boys to make a junior stand in the cold plunge bath whilst they played the hose on him for up to fifteen minutes. It was quite a painful experience.

On that first morning we arrived early to queue outside the dining room for breakfast. On the way down we met 'The Chief', clad in his academic gown which made him look very imposing. He was wont to stand at the top of the stairs and inspect ears and shoes of any new boys. Woe betide anyone found wanting! We were all very overawed, as he knew each individual boy by name even at that early stage.

As we queued up outside the dining room under the supervision of the prefects, one of them was walking along the line taking the names of all the new arrivals. He stopped, looked at me and said, "I know you. You are Ned Stuart's little brother so we shall call you Ned III. Come to think of it. I don't have a fag this year. You appear to be a big strong lad, but a bit thick like your brothers. I think that I could make something out of you. Report to my room at four p.m. It's on the way to the 'Gods'! Don't be late or I'll have your guts for garters!"

"Thank you," I said, for want of something to say. "I won't be late. Where is 'The Gods'?" His reply was terse, "This is your first initiative test. Find out and don't be late!"

My first day at school was very confusing. I didn't know any of the room numbers or who my class mates were so most of us milled around like lost sheep until we found our bearings. I was in a newly-formed group called class 3S, that could mean almost anything from Special to Stupid – certainly not superior. We were a mixed bunch, coming from all sorts of backgrounds, colonial tea planters to local farmers! We spent much of our time collecting stationery, textbooks and getting to know our teachers. Our day finished at 3.30 p.m., when we were free until tea time bell at 5p.m.

After a few enquiries I found the way to the "Gods" and arrived at the prefect's room at 4 p.m.. The door opened at my knock and my fag master appeared. "Come in and first of all meet Denis Hegan who has the bottom bunk. If his fag is not around you will be next in line to help him out. You are very lucky not to be fagging in North dorm where there is a lot of bullying.

"My name is Ted Wilson. I'll show you just what your duties are. Do the job properly and you will keep out of trouble. Here's my locker with clothes and shoes. My rugger kit is in the corner. Your job is to make my bed each morning and keep my shoes polished. Lay out clothes for me to go down town every Friday and Saturday and keep my rugger kit clean and dry for each match. "Have you ever dubbined boots before? If not, get someone to show you! I'm hooker for the first fifteen this year and could be selected to play for Ulster. I shall want my bootlaces blanco'd for important matches and if my kit isn't immaculate I'll kick your arse"

I quickly found out that there is no better teacher than practical experience. In some ways the next few weeks were a bit of a nightmare. Derek was my main tutor as he had undergone a similar experience in the previous year. I spent much of my spare time during the next week trying to soften Ted's rugger boots with dubbin. They had gone very hard since the last season and needed a lot of elbow grease to make them any way normal.

I was acquiring a knack of polishing shoes after a few complaints that I had left polish inside and spoiled his socks. As a result, I was also becoming fairly competent at washing socks. The rugger gear was a never ending chore of scrubbing and cleaning, which gave me those red, cracked hands, so hated by housewives. All the laces had to be taken out of the boots each time, washed, dried and rethreaded. A fag's life was never done! One of my greatest problems was to dry the clothing afterwards. There were no official drying facilities so we made do as best we could. If we found the boiler room open we would string up a makeshift clothes line, otherwise we hung rugby kit in the toilets to dry.

I suffered a couple of beatings with a slipper before half term, mainly for my complete lack of punctuality and inefficiency. I feel that I must have been an awful burden to Ted.

However, I discovered Ted's 'Achilles Heel' early on in our roller coaster relationship. The unfortunate fellow was madly in love with my sister, who was a prefect in the Coleraine High School. In true brotherly fashion, I felt that anyone who loved my red-haired elder sister had to be either lacking in taste or common sense!

I found out that he concealed my sister's photograph beneath his pillow. At this juncture I knew that he must be slightly demented so I would tenderly place the photo on top of his pillow for all the world to see. This indiscipline resulted in a beating with electric light flex!

Sixth formers could go into town on Friday and Saturday afternoons where they had assignations in the local milk bar with girls from the High School. As a fag I had to lay out Ted's clothes on the bed so that he could strut off into town to impress my sister with his elegance. It did not take me long to learn that he was also colour blind, so I arranged some quite striking colour combinations for him. My next beating was with rubber bunsen burner tubing! That hurt!

I must have been either extremely mischievous or slow to learn as I recall that I was beaten at least three times a week during my first year at school. Canes, knotted flex and railway window straps were all used at some time or other. But, not a word to mother that her baby son was having problems!

Chapter Nine

COLERAINE "INST" WAS a school with a long history of academic and sporting achievement. Like my brothers and I, many of the pupils were third generation at the school which, in many ways, gave it a family feeling. Certainly, this fact bound us together as a competitive group at rugby, rowing and cricket against other Ulster schools.

This feeling of unity was backed by the presence of a strong headmaster, 'The Chief,' and several other masters of long standing. Of necessity we had lost several good teachers who had volunteered for military service and these had been replaced by retired or less able teachers.

One of the masters who did worry me at first had long passed his sell-by date. His immediate remedy for any misdemeanour was a clout on the head whilst holding the bowl of his pipe in his hand. He did not last very long so I assumed that a complaint had been laid against him or that he had died of old age.

Teaching staff had to be capable and strong with ninety boys locked into a boarding school system. In retrospect, the boarding experience was an excellent training ground for boys, like myself, who were lacking in self-discipline.

We had several boarding staff who had rooms above the South and Middle dorms. They varied in their ability to control the boys from quite strict to hopeless.

'Whip' Cordner was really too nice and friendly to be a schoolmaster. Unfortunately, his vision was terribly poor and he wore very thick spectacles. As a disciplinarian he was hopeless and consequently everyone took advantage of him. Life must have been very miserable for him at times as he knew that he could not control a class and so did the boys.

He would turn round from the blackboard to find a flight of paper aeroplanes flying across the room or somebody would flick a lighted match into the waste paper basket to cause a bit of distraction. Of course he would not see it until it was well alight.

The star stunt in his class was when one of the day boys would throw a packet of sandwiches across the room to a boarding friend. Whip would see the sandwiches in the air but not the hand that shot up and grabbed them, so his eyes followed the line of flight after they had vanished.

His one outstanding achievement, however, was his ability to construct cat's whisker radio sets. At this he excelled and had developed his set to receive Lord Haw-Haw, the Nazi propagandist who used to broadcast from Berlin. None of the boys at school could emulate this feat.

At bath night, the boarding masters would walk through our dormitory to reach their bathroom, turn on the bath tap and then head back to their room to change. After five minutes they could return, clad in dressing gowns, to a bath full of hot water.

This system worked very well until one evening, when Whip decided to have a bath. Soon after he turned on the tap, three of us rushed into the bathroom and pulled out the plug. Needless to say, when he returned five minutes later to find the bath empty and ten junior boys sound asleep, he was very cross indeed. We might have got away with it if Billy MacVicker, hiding under the bedclothes had not broken into snorts of suppressed laughter. On went the light and poor Billy was accused of carrying out this criminal act!

It had been a very frustrating term for Whip as he had already suffered at the hands of the sixth formers. At one stage he could not find his bicycle and was unable to see that it had been hoisted onto a hook on the ceiling. A further episode involved him being locked in the lavatory. The thought of junior pupils playing pranks on him was just too much!

Since we had all helped to plan this prank we all insisted that we had pulled out the plug and must share in the punishment. Faced with this act of solidarity Willie ordered us into the boarding staff common room for punishment. We were all lined up in a row and each of us received six strokes of the cane across our pyjama'd bottoms.

The usual series of Billy Bunter sounds such as 'Ooh! Ah!' and " 'Oh sir, that hurts' rent the air. We felt very sorry for him as sixty strokes must have left him with an extremely stiff arm next day. He was so short-sighted that he had not realised that we all had exercise books stuffed down the seats of our pyjamas!

Night time in the South Dorm was always a hive of activity. We would talk and plot for a long time. Midnight feasts were always great adventures at the start of term when we had brought food back from home. We had to choose a night when the masters had gone out and the matron was in charge. We hoped that she would not catch us as she had a deadly aim with a pair of Billy MacVicker's braces, which she had confiscated.

As it grew late, out would come the cakes, chocolates (brought across the border from Eire), tins of beans and sardines, with bread nicked from the kitchens. All this would be laid out under our beds and passed around the dorm from bed to bed. It really was a gala night when we talked about our holiday exploits and fought over our share of the food.

We were disturbed by the matron's arrival a couple of times. Fortunately, our lookout on the stairs gave us an early warning and as she passed through to check the other dormitories there was only the sound of sleeping little cherubs. How on earth she did not smell the food I shall never know! I had to lie motionless in bed one night, with my heel resting in a tin of sardines in tomato sauce, under the bedclothes, whilst she chatted with a prefect at the open door.

Rob Patterson slept at the end of the dormitory beside the wall of the boarding staff common room. Through a crack in the timbered back of his locker it was possible to see into the common room – an ideal vantage point for boys bent on mischief!

One night when the matron was on dormitory duty we realised that the masters had probably gone out together for the evening. Looking through the peephole confirmed this as the table in the common room was laid out for a veritable feast to greet their return. Unable to resist such a good opportunity to have an adventure, we sent out a scouting party to investigate the situation. The report came back that the table was groaning with food so we worked out that with so much sustenance they would probably not miss 10 sausage rolls, a few cup cakes and 10 pieces of wheaten bread.

The best laid plans of mice and men aft times 'gang a'gley.' We sent out a foraging group to gather our victuals and rearrange the plates so that they still looked full. A very fine meal was enjoyed by all after which we went to sleep before the staff returned.

We should have realised next day that everything was progressing too smoothly and lived in the blissful ignorance that we were undetected! Late that night whilst we were fast asleep a number of dark figures crept into our dormitory. I awoke after hot candlewax dropped onto my eyelids, by brother Ted, and simultaneously all our beds were turned upside down. Just as quickly and silently our intruders vanished, leaving us struggling in the dark, to escape from our blankets and turn our beds right side up. Then came the job of making our beds in the dark as drawing the attention of the staff would have found little sympathy.

The news reached us on the grapevine next day that the sixth form dormitory had been blamed for the food escapade and had subsequently been 'gated' on the Friday afternoon. The staff could not accept that the youngsters in South Dorm would get up to such pranks, so the seniors took retribution into their own hands! Life was hard as a junior!

A couple of the sixth-formers that year did exceed their position and enjoyed bullying. One poor young lad, Trout Wallace, who later became a senior officer in the navy, was hung out of a third storey window by his ankles, as a punishment.

Several of us provided sport for the seniors when they became bored on a wet afternoon. We would be summoned to the North Dormitory which contained cubicles. The poor unfortunate junior had to stand in the passage whilst his persecutors skimmed metal plates up and down the passage, trying to hit him.

Fortunately, these incidents were few and far between, and I cannot recall anyone being permanently affected by them, although this rough life could have influenced those few boys who ran away from school. The seniors in the following years certainly seemed to have a much kinder attitude to the younger pupils.

Life at a boarding school could become very humdrum unless you had an interest. I was not particularly keen on rugby at that stage as I still had breathing problems after my T.B. but did turn out about once a week and joined in the running which led out along the Ballycairn Road and returned down the main road, past the Loretto Convent. That was quite exciting as the Loretto girls had the reputation of being sex-starved maidens! Unfortunately they were kept locked away.

Once I learned the rules I played quite a lot of handball on the court behind the chemistry laboratory. Handball is played on a three walled court. The ball in our case was a tennis ball, hit with the hand, and the game resembled a cross between 'fives' and squash. It could be a very energetic occupation. We also played quite a bit of football in Sausage Park, a grassy area between the school and the chemistry laboratory. As in all schools, games went in cycles.

One game that my father played as a boy was called "Tipcat". This involved placing a stick at an angle across a stone and hitting it with a second stick so that it flew up in the air. As it rotated in the air, the striking stick was used to hit it away as far as possible.

Many of the rainy days meant that we were all crammed indoors or in our dormitories. In the common room we could play table tennis or use the same table to play a variation on 'shove ha'penny' adapted to football.

"Churchies" was another wet weather game where we would select two teams. One member of the team would stand, as the church spire, back to a wall, whilst the first member would put their head between his legs and grasp his thighs and so on until all the team formed a crocodile with heads between the legs of the boy in front. The object of the game was for the second team to leap frog over the rear of the crocodile and land as far up as possible until their weight caused the crocodile to collapse.

We used to spend hours at this game despite its dangers. Because I was well built I excelled at this sport, although I did end up in hospital as a result, having been kicked severely. There was also a lot of time spent on less arduous activities such as reading, stamp-collecting, and constructing our own illegal radios.

We were always thinking up new ideas for leisure time. I ran a tombola for a ten-shilling note and made a pound. Brother Derek was very gifted and each term he would make money by writing poems or short stories for the school magazine and selling them.

Food restrictions were fairly severe during the war years and we all had to present our ration books to the matron at the start of term. Despite the food scarcity, the staff tried hard to feed us a nutritious diet. Boiled potatoes were a staple diet and, after I expressed a liking for potato skins, I would have my plate piled full each day. The vegetables were set out in dishes along the table, although we did find that over-boiled soggy cabbage every day was a bit boring. To make life interesting one day, I arranged to have a matchstick stuck into each cabbage dish bearing a notice – 'Please keep off the Grass.' I felt that it was a bit unreasonable when the matron hit me! Other staple dishes were porridge for breakfast and rice pudding for dinner – very nutritious food, which often contained added protein in the way of maggots and moths! Eggs only appeared on Sunday mornings.

There were often fried breakfasts during the week, which was appropriate for youngsters expending a lot of energy. It could vary between fried bacon or spam accompanied by fried bread. Now the fried bread itself was soggy and greasy enough, but when the light blew out in the oven and the fat was full of coal gas it added that extra piquancy to the meal!

Early on I developed a reputation for losing my keys and, of necessity, I had to become an efficient lock picker in order to get into my locker for clothes and rugger kit. After a period my skills as a cracks-man were in demand for other less gifted pupils.

I think that my greatest achievement was to be able to open the caretaker's cupboard using only a pair of dividers. This was pure delight as it contained duplicate keys for the whole school. As a result, a chosen group would disappear downstairs at night, use the keys to enter the pantry which supplied bread, butter and jam. Then we went off to the boiler room which was always warm and cozy and seated in front of the boiler we could have jam and toast as well as talking into the early hours.

Once we moved up into "The Gods", which was reasonably isolated from the staff room and the other dormitories, these keys gave us access to the A.T.C. room which contained a loudspeaker. When this was connected up to one of the hidden radios we could have music all night.

One light summer's evening, about 10 p.m., the radio was blasting, the air was blue with cigarette smoke and one of my friends was leaning out of the window with a .22 air rifle, shooting rats down below in the sergeant's hen run. Suddenly, in came Sam Lyons, one of the boarding masters who played rugby in town and enjoyed a few beers. He walked up the dormitory, confiscated the gun and walked out again. We were speechless as he did not comment on any of our other transgressions.

Needless to say, we could not lose a good .22 rifle so a search party was sent off to retrieve it, in the dead of night. Sam had gone off to bed to sleep off the effects of a good night at the rugby club and left the gun resting alongside the mantlepiece in the boarding staff room. Never at a loss, the culprits replaced the gun with a Boer War drill carbine "borrowed" from the Army Cadet hut!

Next morning Sam was seen to be wandering around with the carbine in his hand, wondering how it came into his possession as it was incapable of firing anything! Part of his confusion was put down to a king-size hangover.

At the start of each rugby season all the keen boys would be seen out practising and exercising muscles which had lain dormant during the summer. These stalwarts could be seen hobbling around for a few days. To ease the aching muscles they would buy a bottle of Sloan's liniment and rub it into the aching thighs. 'The best laid plans of mice and men!' applied as we had the odd boy who overdid the application and had to spend several hours sitting in the wash basin to cool his burning scrotum.

None of the staff, except the 'Chief,' were immune from the machinations of the pupils. The last day of the school year was always the time for retribution by those boys who, rightly or wrongly, felt that they had been put upon or perhaps punished just a result of high spirits when retribution was impossible.

Normally, the staff would see the boys off the premises before they, in turn, departed. Supervising cases and trunks en route to the railway station started early in the day, followed by the sergeant and teachers walking around the dormitories and classrooms to check for articles carelessly left behind or illicitly removed.

Late in the afternoon, Sammy Lyons prepared to leave on his motorbike and drive home to Ballycastle. He was greatly dismayed to find that his beloved BSA Bantam appeared to have left before him. He searched high and low but it remained painfully evident by its absence. At length Sam resigned himself to another night at school in order to continue the hunt next day.

Surprise! Surprise! When he returned to his bedroom, there was his cherished little bike, cosily tucked up in his bed. Unfortunately, it was somewhat incontinent and there was a black pool of oil on the sheets. History must have recorded his comments, but I had left school by that time! Sam's humiliation was complete when he met 'the Chief' and the matron on the stairs as he wheeled his bike down the stairs. I should imagine that he had a problem explaining away the large pool of oil in his bed.

This was the final fling of a particularly spirited year. Some weeks earlier we had held a most enjoyable sports day. The sun reigned resplendent in an azure sky. The sergeant had spent some time, with the groundsman, marking out the running track and siting the various events, and the boys had spent many hours in training for the cherished Victor Ludorum shield.

I even qualified for the high jump, although I could not compete with those who used the Western Roll, and finished in seventh place. At lunch time the school grounds started to fill up with spectators. Mums dressed in large brimmed hats and dresses with dads in sports jackets or blazers. Of course, the younger members of the family turned up to see big brothers competing for honours and elder sisters were under scrutiny from talent spotting boarders. Tea and sandwiches were served on the upper lawn in front of the headmaster's office, where it was beautifully shaded by the row of mature elms.

All of the staff were running hither and thither to help to organise the day's proceedings and escort parents on guided tours of the school and dormitories, which had been spruced up earlier in the day under the brooding supervision of the sergeant, who insisted that all the beds were made neatly and in military style.

All went according to plan and the spectators drifted away after a very pleasant day when the time came for the staff to head homewards. "Banjo" MacCauley, a very popular mathematics teacher was ready to leave when he found that his Morris 8 was missing.

At this he became quite irascible, as it had been a long, hot day and he was very tired. Gathering a squad of boys together he sent them in all directions in search of his vehicle and it was about three-quarters-of-an-hour later that it was found, locked in the gymnasium. Nothing further was said but he was quite suspicious of the Portstewart boys, particularly Knox and Fawcett, who were his neighbours.

As boys we always seized the opportunity to exploit the weaknesses or idiosyncrasies of the staff. One of our wartime staff was 'Pips' Wheeler, a retired army officer, who had a strong affinity to spiritual refreshment. In the classroom he would regularly disappear behind the uplifted lid of his desk or leave us some set work whilst he headed to the toilet for medicinal purposes! He must have been a very competent tutor as he raised my maths level from "dunce" to the top third of the class within twelve months. I have always been intrigued by the effect that a teacher can have on an individual pupil. With his gift of teaching he left me with a passion for algebra and trigonometry.

Pip took time off for illness and in the interregnum we had a new graduate, Miss Mary McPherson, immediately christened 'Bitchy'. An ex-wren, she was tough and a good teacher, but she started off with the disadvantage of being the only female member of staff. At this time there was an entrenched belief that women stayed at home and brought up the children. No self-respecting Ulsterman would be seen pushing a pram!

Rafferty's Law applied to teaching in that, no matter how many blackboard rubbers you supplied, there was never one available when needed. Mary managed to disguise her well-rounded figure from the eyes of lusting and macho young adolescents beneath an academic gown. I think, without exception, we were all in love with this comely maiden. She had a habit of wiping the blackboard with the tail of her gown which concurrently lifted her skirt above those delectable knees and ruined our concentration. It was some time before she discovered that, boys being boys, someone had placed a mirror on the floor under her desk.

Across the corridor from the maths room was Gordon Mahoney's classroom. He was a mountain of a man, with features hewn out of granite and topped with tightly-curled and grizzled hair. He and his twin brother had once played in the Irish rugby pack. An awe-inspiring sight!

In class he lived and breathed everyday life in Rome, and any pupil who was not inspired by "De Bello Gallico" or the translation of Ovid was in deep trouble. He had started his teaching career with a new academic gown which over the years had become green and torn in strips, which trailed behind as he walked down the corridor. Each strip was lovingly knotted to prevent further deterioration. In retrospect, the gown (or what was left of it) looked silly on his giant shambling frame. He would stand at the front of the class expecting each boy to be word perfect in declensions and tenses, and when we stammered out an imperfect reply he would roar out, in despair, "Oh! Don't you see sonny. This will never get you through your examinations in June."

When he set us work to do in class it was a brave boy who doodled or gazed about. He would walk up and down slowly between the rows of desks and any boy found wanting received encouragement as an arm would swing and a set of clenched knuckles caught the unfortunate victim on the back of the head, lifting him up in the air. A less severe crime would only warrant being lifted up by the ear. His enthusiasm carried me along and, despite my lack of academic prowess, I enjoyed his living Latin – so much so that I had a second try when I failed my junior latin examination.

At the end of the corridor was the geography room where 'Pansy' Magrath and Sammy Lyons were in charge. We had always understood that Pansy was a handball champion although I never saw him in action. On one particular day I was feeling particularly bored and could not concentrate on academia as Pansy was pacing up and down with a flapping sole on his shoe-very distracting for keen academics.

It was all fair game for a chuckle, as he became more and more embarrassed, pretending to ignore his gait, which became increasingly like that of a penguin. I was watching my pal, Barney Streether, drawing rapid cartoons of current affairs, such as Pansy's sole, Hitler, and Spitfires shooting down an overfed Hermann Goering, in his Messerschmidt 109.

Chapter Ten

I HAD BEEN INVOLVED in thinking of higher things, as I gazed out of the classroom window, across the playground, affectionately called Sausage Park, towards the chemistry and physics laboratories, and beyond. Even at that age, I knew what I didn't want to do when I grew up.

I definitely didn't want to be an engineer, probably because I had never been interested in being a train driver when I was little. Anyway the trains in the Isle of Man, where I had grown up, were very small themselves! Carpentry was out as I couldn't hold a chisel! I was no good at sports and I decidedly did not want to be a doctor like my dad, as they had to work awfully hard and had ghastly children.

Problems of this sort weigh heavily on the mind, when you are 13 years old and not very deeply committed to a career. I liked the idea of medicine, but there were too many fat ladies and crippled old men to deal with all the time! My great passion as a little boy, apart from being a beachcomber, which was romantic, but didn't pay much, was to be a zoo keeper. Often, I had thought of a life with elephants and tigers, but there really were not too many zoos to work in!

The next best thing was to be a farmer, with fields all around me, and I could have horses, cows and pigs to look after. As I was gazing out through the rain-streaked window, Iwatched a farmer, driving his grey Ford-Ferguson tractor across a potato field. He had a sack draped over his back to keep the torrential rain at bay and another over his legs for protection. That sight was burnt into my mind and farming immediately was pigeonholed in the "didn't want to do" section. There was only one option left, and that was to become a vet. The problem was that I didn't know much about being a vet!

I thought about this problem for a few days, because no one amongst my friends could help me. On Saturday afternoon, after playing rugby in the morning, we were given a pass to go into the town. If we were silly enough to have been detected in any unauthorised activities during the previous week, we were "gated" and no pass was issued.

I had to be particularly smart, as a visit into town meant oven-fresh soda farls and fadge (Irish potato bread), at my grandparents' house. I would rush into the house to see old Lizzie, the cook, who sat me down at the scrubbed kitchen table and plied me with warm sodas, butter and strawberry jam. Those were times of great ecstasy for Derek and me, and then we would go into the front room to see my grandparents.

I can still see the house in my mind's eye, as a splendid double fronted, Victorian house of the type occupied by genteel business folk. It was situated on a side road and looked out across the river. An imposing, rather than beautiful, building, grey in colour with a sizeable front door embellished by a large black knocker.

Opening off from the main hallway were two large rooms, dining -room on the left and sitting-room on the right side. The dining-room contained a highly polished table, to seat eight people, and a matching sideboard, which contained the silver. Sunday teas were the highlight of the week at this great table on which I once counted thirteen different types of bread. The most exciting part of the meal was to see which of the children, in gran's judgement, had been the best behaved during the meal. To that fortunate child was given the privilege of licking the jam spoon.

On the other side of the hallway was the drawing-room, where my grandparents and aunt spent much of their time. It had a timeless air, the damask covered suite, china display cabinet and paintings of Highland cattle gave it an atmosphere of its own. Instead of a grandfather clock, there was a brass clock, under a glass dome, with four brass balls, which gyrated back and forth. I spent many hours trying to find out how it worked, I'm still not sure!

Like so many rooms of that era, before central heating, a heavy curtain hung across the door to keep out draughts. This was further reinforced by an extending leather screen, covered with lines of brass studs.

My grandmother, who was extremely religious, spent her day reading missals and prayers. She was a very dignified old lady, always dressed in black, with a lacy mob cap. Encircling her throat was a plain band of black velvet or, when she was feeling particularly skittish, the band would be purple. Her quiet words of wisdom keep returning to me, as in later years I realised the effect that she had had on my life!

My grandfather, on the other hand, was a first-rate business man and, unlike many in those days, he treated everyone equally, irrespective of class or creed. Immaculately dressed, in a smart grey suit, and sporting a handlebar moustache, he cut an imposing figure. He got along very well with people, and had the Ulsterman's work ethic, which helped him to progress from draper's apprentice to the owner of a very successful garage business which was continued by his son, Graham, for many years.

His acute sense of humour was an outstanding feature which endeared him to us, as children. Graham was like my grandfather and shared his zest for work. He enjoyed company and always arrived in after Sunday tea to tell us all the latest news and funny stories.

Chapter Eleven

WHEN I ARRIVED at the house that weekend, I told my aunt of my momentous decision to be a vet and, without hesitation, she sent me in to see John and Jack Morrow, who were in veterinary practice next door. They took to me right away, as they had no children, and from that day onwards, all my spare time at weekends was spent in their dispensary, or in the kitchen, listening intently, to tales of horses with Monday Morning Leg, cows with gargot and sheep with worms. All these strange names opened up a new world to my young brain.

In retrospect, they epitomised the art of veterinary practice; the ability to deal with a client in a manner which gained his utmost respect and still kept one's skills cloaked in an aura of mystery. I was very lucky as many boys at that time had to pay a premium to learn in a veterinary practice. Jack would tell me of the gold medals that he gained at veterinary college, and I wondered if I should ever reach such heights – I didn't!

Best of all, was the veterinary dispensary, with its great mahogany benches and shelves, two sinks, a couple of pestles and mortars and a set of scales. This was the centre of operations, as most drugs at that time were administered by mouth. Virtually the only injectable drugs were sulphadimidine and prontosil, precursors to the penicillins and streptomycin of later years. Prontosil had the added enhancement of turning the urine red; which from the farmers point of view showed that it must be doing good!

My sterling qualities, as an unpaid lackey, were soon realised, and John set to work to educate me in dispensing. When they were at work, the housekeeper, Miss Hunter, oversaw my training. I was so keen that I quickly became half proficient. I would make up drenches for cattle, balls for horses and lots of powders. These all had to be prepared very accurately, weighed out, added to liquids, or in the case of electuaries, mixed with molasses. I had to learn to measure drugs in grains, drachms and minims, which I had never met before.

The walls were lined with large bottles, called Winchester quarts, carrying labels with Latin names, such as Spirits Ammon. Aromat., Ol. Terebinth, Liq. Ammon. Forte and many more exotic sounding names.

Underneath the bottles were rows of square ended drawers, with such titles as Pulv. Zingib., Pulv. Nux Vom. Gentian and Pulv Catechu, to mention but a few. My curiosity knew no bounds, as I wandered along the shelves, pondering on the uses of the drugs. I did not realise at that stage, that veterinary science had me hooked for life.

All the medicinal compounds were kept in a recipe book. All the prescriptions written out in beautiful copperplate script. All weights and measures were entered with extraordinary accuracy, as many of these drugs were acutely poisonous in overdosage. These were regarded as very confidential, and never to be conveyed to neighbouring practices.

During quiet periods in the practice we would set to, making up medicines. Two big piles of paper, one white the other brown, would be laid on the bench. They were all cut to a certain size to suit the medicine containers.

Beside these, with military precision, were laid out a series of labels, sealing wax, bunsen burner and string. As each liquid medicine was prepared, bottled and corked, it was then passed along to be very neatly wrapped in paper, both ends were sealed with red sealing wax and another label stuck on the outside. Powdered medicines were weighed out (in drachms and grains) either put in a box, as one dose, or if for a series of doses, would be folded neatly into little packets sealed with hot sealing wax.

After about thirty of these packets were prepared they were then placed on brown paper. Medicines were then put into rows, in a glass-fronted cabinet, for sale to the farmers. For small animal clients we had a pill making machine which eased the labour of making tablets. One of my jobs was to mix powders together by grinding them with a pestle and mortar.

It is well to remember that in those times there were no antibiotics available and now we have reached the stage of antibiotic resistance across the world. Where did we go wrong?

Jack and John were good tutors. I was sometimes allowed to go on the farm calls with them. On my first trip, we were driving along a country track in his battered Ford Popular, when Jack grabbed a handful of grass from the hedge, and presented them to me. "How many different types of grass can you see there, Boy?" I took a deep breath because grass was only a plant that grew in fields.

"Come on," he said," All cows eat grass, and it is up to you to know which grasses are good or poor feed. Sort them out, and I will tell you each one, and the next time I'll test you, until you know them all."

Vets in those days were not versed in biochemistry and pathology to such a high degree, but they had a great knowledge of basic stockmanship and animal husbandry. Part of our problem nowadays is that we have to absorb so much advanced information, that we cannot put it across to the farmer in terms which he understands. As we are crammed with more and more technical information, it becomes increasingly difficult for young graduates to talk the same language as their clients.

I went out with John to a holding of some ten cows. One of the cows had blood in her milk. We entered the low cow byre, smelling of warm cattle and sweet hay. The cows were chained up in pairs and it was hard to squeeze up in between them. A couple of chickens scuttled out the door past us, whilst a third clucked contentedly that she had laid an egg in the corner, on some hay.

John examined the cow closely, and found a bruise on the udder where she had been fighting. As he looked at her and chatted to the farmer, he leaned back against the neighbouring animal. As he stepped out from between the cows he turned to the farmer and said "Yon beast should have a fine calf within six weeks, and I'll lay odds that she milks well for you." The farmer was left scratching his head as to how Mr Morrow, who hadn't even looked at the beast, could tell him so much about her. "Easy," chuckled John on the way home, "as I was leaning against her, the calf kicked me in the back, and I rolled her skin between my fingers and it felt very fine – the sign of a good milker." That is what we call the veterinary art.

One afternoon I was tidying up the dispensary area, when Jack arrived in from a call. He called to me, saying, "Boy, here's some money, go on up to the tobacconist on the corner of the bridge and buy me an ounce of plug tobacco." I must have looked a bit quizzical, as no one in the house smoked cigarettes, let alone a pipe. I don't suppose that it was very common for a 13-year-old to ask for an ounce of pipe tobacco either.

I duly returned with my purchase. Jack presented me with a penknife and paper with instructions to cut it up into thin slices and then put it into the oven for a couple of hours. I was agog with curiosity at this new turn of events but resolved to be patient and not ask questions.

Later that afternoon I was allowed to remove the dried out tobacco to the dispensary where it was ground to a powder with the pestle and mortar.

"Thank you," said Jack, "now fetch me the recipe book and we can add some bluestone to it make up some worm drenches for cattle. We must be sure to use exact quantities, as an overdose can be very poisonous. Don't you dare to tell other people about our preparation."

I used to watch, with great fascination, the manner in which medicines were administered to animals. It was not always the size of the operator that counted, but the knack of administration. Most drugs were given by mouth, which required manpower to restrain the animal. In those days farming was labour intensive with many of the workers living in "tied" cottages. These were provided free or at a minimal rent provided that the tenant was an employee of the owner. Consequently we were never short of helping hands.

The ideal situation with horses was to give medicines in food or water. Unfortunately many drugs were unpalatable and had to be given as a ball or an electuary.

Horse balls were often given as a physic or purge and consisted of aloes, glycerine, hard soap, beeswax and other additives. The constituents were melted down, allowed to set, weighed out and then rolled into cylinders about three inches long. Many horsemen carried their own balling guns and would administer them very efficiently.

The balling gun consisted of a hollow rod with a cup at one end, for holding the ball, and a central plunger for expelling it over the back of the horse's tongue. To use the gun, a gag could be inserted in the horse's mouth to keep the mouth open. Alternatively, a skilled operator could grasp the horse's tongue firmly in his hand and rotate his fist, in front of the cheek teeth, to form a gag which prevented a horse from closing his mouth. In this manner the other hand was free to use the balling gun. The same technique is used when using a dental "float" to rasp a horse's teeth.

Electuaries, which are still in use, consist of the medication mixed well with thick treacle. This is given on a flat, spatula-shaped stick which is pulled across the tongue and cheek teeth of the horse. The molasses is so sticky that it remains in the mouth and tastes quite pleasant.

Rubber or plastic tubing is probably the most efficient method of ensuring that all liquid medicines go down to the stomach and consists of passing a long rubber tube, with a rounded tip, up the horses nostril so that it rests at the back of the throat. The intention is that, on feeling the tube, the patient will automatically swallow the end of the tube and it will pass into the gullet from whence it may be pushed gently into the stomach, and the liquid may be poured into the other end via a funnel. It is possible to watch the tube passing down the gullet as it lies close to the skin. This technique was described to us at college as a simple and straightforward operation. In retrospect I feel that the college horses must have been trained to swallow the tubes as it was very simple when under instruction.

Disasters beset my first feeble attempts. Either the tube was too big or went up the wrong passage, in the nostril, causing intensive bleeding which did not impress the owners one bit although it didn't concern the horses. One tube was too fine and bent so that the horse chewed the end with his back teeth whilst another was so stiff that it went down the windpipe where he could have drowned if any liquid had been poured down. We were taught to shake the windpipe and a misdirected tube would then be heard to rattle. The height of bliss for a young vet is to be able to watch and feel the tube sliding down the gullet or watch its progress down the neck.

Many times I have been called upon to drench a horse using a long necked wine bottle. Drenching is a skilled technique at the best of times. Pouring liquid down an animal's throat would seem to be a fairly simple procedure until you try it yourself. The patient has an innate aversion to having nasty tasting medicine poured down its throat, particularly if you have a firm hold on its nose or tongue. I have always held cattle by the jaw and worked their tongue with my fingers to make them swallow whilst I slowly pour in the drench, lest they choke on it.

Now, a horse is taller and much more flighty. Not only that, but he contrives to hold the drench at the back of his throat, under his tongue and inside his lips so that when you are walking away with a satisfied smile, he snorts large quantities of linseed oil and turpentine over your head, face and any clothing which you are wearing.

I was helping John Morrow clean out his stables one day when he warned me not to go through one door as there was a dog called Rufus inside. Rufus was a very overweight labrador who lived in a pub. Rufus's amiable nature was his downfall. He was inclined to greet all the clients as they entered and spent many happy hours hoovering up discarded potato crisps which increased his stature. The dog's owners had gone away for two weeks and left the dog with John as it was overweight. I knew very little about slimming dogs and was interested in the slimming diet.

"Well," said John," You must realise that many dogs reflect their owners who are either too old or too lazy to exercise them. It's rather like stoking an engine. All the fuel or food has to be burnt up as energy used in exercise or keeping warm. If it isn't then the energy is converted into fat and he puts on weight and starts scratching – just like you when you get heat spots from eating too many cornflakes."

I could understand this explanation. "But how do you slim them?" I asked, as I had not seen him out walking a dog on a lead.

"Aye, that's a good question," he said, tilting his hat back on his head. "This wee dog comes in every year, very overweight. I stop all his biscuit and replace it with raw vegetables- chopped up carrots, cabbage and the like. They are over ninety per cent water and make him feel full without much energy going in. I generally leave the meat part of the meal as it is. When they come back in two weeks their wee fat dog will be a lot thinner and leaping about all over the place. They'll never change in spite of me telling them that he's overfed. He'll be back next year"

"Some people are strange about their pets and over-indulge them, rather as happens with many only children, instead of a skelp across the backside at the right time. All young animals are more contented if they live within well-defined boundaries. Just you wait and see what happens next week when Rex arrives for a stay." With this little homily, John jumped into his car and drove off into the town.

Some weeks later I had just returned from a call with John, when Rex arrived with his owner who was just departing on holiday. I had never seen such a large and mean looking Alsatian. He arrived already muzzled, towing his owner, Mike McCartney, behind him.

On seeing John and I a deep rumble started off somewhere in his chest, terminating as a snarl and revealing a set of wicked looking yellow fangs.

Mike smiling, said, "Here you are, John. I slipped on his muzzle as I knew that he'd have a go at you. I'm the only one in the family that can handle him. Indeed, I was quite worried this morning as he held my son in the corner and wouldn't let him move. When we get back we shall have to sort him out."

"Right," responded John, "Just you leave him in the loose-box here. Take his muzzle off and shut him in. I've left him a good straw bed and plenty of water inside. By the time you come back we should have come to terms."

Turning to me, he said, "Now don't you go in there by yourself, Noel. Rex can be very dangerous until he settles down. Come in at five o'clock and watch me feed him."

When five o'clock came around John mixed him some meat and biscuit in a bowl and told me to stand well back. As he opened the loose-box door a couple of inches, there was a roar from inside as Rex, in full snarl, hurled himself at the opening. Quickly, John slammed and bolted the door, and with the bowl in his hand said, "There you are now, I don't think Rex is very hungry tonight. Maybe he'll have learnt some manners by the morning. In the meantime, my labrador will be pleased to scoff this lot."

I called in the next evening to find that Rex had repeated his attack in the morning despite being hungry. As John brought his meal across, he kept talking to him quietly, and gently opened the door Rex grumbled and grizzled from the middle of the loose-box so John left him a handful of food inside before closing the door.

"He's getting quite hungry now so I'll throw him in some more several times this evening. Eventually he'll realise that I am the source of food and will appreciate my coming. I shall also dominate him by making him sit until he is allowed to eat. A dog's natural instinct is to become pack leader and unless he is dominated by his owners he will assert his "Top Dog" position. Any challenge to his authority will be met with aggression or marking his territory in the house by cocking his leg on the furniture."

Within four days, Rex assumed his subordinate position and was well fed and happy at the bottom of the pecking order, so I was able to take over the feeding. He then had the impertinence to defend us against his master when he returned. A few strong words from John reinforced the necessity for the rest of the family to take part in the feeding and discipline of Rex He came to see us many times after that and we never had to resort to a muzzle.

During the war years, horses were still being used extensively for everyday work on the farm. As they were indispensable, the vet was called in as soon as any problems arose. Tractors were few and far between and fuel scarce. It was no surprise when Rob McNulty, who had a small farm out beyond Moneycarrey schoolhouse, dropped in on the market day and asked John to pay him a visit in the evening to see a lame Clydesdale colt that he had just broken in.

"Are you comin' for a wee run in the car?" asked John when I called in after teatime. "We'll go and have a look at this horse of Rob's." He could not have chosen a worse autumn night.

It was blowing a hooley and the rain was coming down in sheets as we drove off in his battered little Ford Popular. The pale glow of the street lamps in Coleraine appeared quite subdued by the storm and people were standing, sheltering in shop doorways, with coat collars buttoned up against the weather.

It was freezing cold in the car as the heating system in that model was remarkable for its inefficiency. We did not say much as the little car fought its way up the narrow hill against the rivers of water cascading down the road. The windows misted over, requiring constant clearing as the wipers struggled to clear the torrents pouring down the glass.

On reaching the level, we gradually increased speed along a straight stretch of road and as we rushed over the cross roads a side wind picked the car up, like a rag doll, and landed us on the grass verge on the right side of the road. I suppose that we were fortunate that there was no traffic coming the other way or trees on the grass, as John clung firmly onto the steering wheel, staring fixedly ahead as he pulled us back onto the correct side of the road.

"It's a wild old night," he said laconically, "There won't be many courting couples about tonight. Thirty years ago my Da' would have done this journey with a pony and trap and ended up at the farm well-nigh soaked. Mind you, there would have been a good meal waiting for him and a bed for the night."

We slowed up beside a little white cottage at the roadside and turned into a small cobbled yard beside the house. Almost as soon as we drove in, the backdoor opened and a jumble of figures stumbled out into the night.

By the light of a hurricane lamp we found our way across the yard and entered the stable. It was fairly small inside, with only a couple of stalls and space for the harness and feed bins. The low roof space created by the barn floor above made it appear even more cramped.

Robbie said, "You'll have met my two neighbours perhaps, Mr Morrow? They've come to assist you. Here's Willie John Patterson who you met last summer on that case of gargot in his best cow, and David McFeeter who has just arrived in from Ballycastle. They are both good men with a horse."

John nodded and acknowledged both men. He had known Willie John and his father for many years. He had no great liking for either father or son. They were both big, red-faced men who ran smallholdings in the area and did a bit of dealing as a sideline. Much of their time was spent at the weekly markets, buying and selling cattle and ponies.

They both drank too much and rolled home many times in such a state that they had no control over their charges. At such times they drove their horse so hard that on a couple of occasions the horse panicked, tipping trap and passengers into the ditch. Rogues of the highest order, they were up to all the tricks of the trade in horse dealing, rasping teeth, dumping toes and many other techniques to pass off an unsound animal as a good bargain, to the unwary purchaser.

"Thanks Robbie," said John, "If you would like to take his head I shall have a look at the colt." He moved over towards the large Clydesdale in the stall who was holding a hind leg in the air, toe just touching the ground. Gently sliding his hand down the leg from the stifle to the hock joint he felt the muscles and joints. Talking to the animal all the time, to give it confidence, his hand quietly moved towards the heel until the colt, Prince, flinched and raised his leg in pain.

"He has some swelling in the coronet and pastern, possibly coming from the foot. Robbie, could you get a pail of hot water from the house and another lamp so that we can see a bit better," commented John.

As Rob disappeared out of the door, David took over duty, holding Prince's head collar whilst John got out his foot knife and started to trim away the sole of the foot, removing any mud and dung in the process.

"Look here," continued John, as his knife struck something solid, "I've found the problem. Bring the light a wee bit nearer and you will see a nail sticking into the sole of his foot." Levering it out he held a hob nail in the palm of his hand.

As Rob returned with a pail of hot water and a Tilley lamp John said "There you are now. There's your culprit and it has taken a bit of infection in with it. Look at that nasty grey, stinking muck pouring out of the hole. I'll just pare it back a wee bit to give good drainage then with a poultice and some serum to protect against tetanus he should recover fairly quickly."

All the men were leaning forward to watch the operation. When John's knife touched a tender spot, Prince's leg shot out like a powerful piston, knocking Willie John into the corner beside the feed bin. The hurricane lamp shot in the air and the glass shattered at my feet. Some oil spilled out onto a patch of straw which started to burn and there was general pandemonium as the flames spread. By the light of the Tilley lamp David picked up the pail of water and poured it over the burning straw, washing any loose oil into the drain.

John strode across and helped Willie John to his feet, none the worse for his tumble. "Sorry, Rob," said John, chuckling, "No need to call the fire engine. We seem to be a bit short of water for the poultice. Can you bring some old rags and oilskin back with you."

When the hot water arrived, John said to me, "Now watch this. Hand me over that iodoform powder. It's a disinfectant." Taking some of the powder he poured it into the hole in the horses foot and a puff of purple smoke stood out against the light from the Tilley lamp. There was a gasp of astonishment from the farmers, who felt that a demonstration of this sort meant that the drug must be very effective.

"Get me some bran and Epsom salts and wrap them up in that clean rag, Noel. Screw it up and I shall dip it into the pail of hot water to make a poultice. Rob, lift a foreleg to stop him kicking and I shall put it onto the foot, like that, cover it with oilcloth and wrap it up in the corner of a sack. Now, tie it above the fetlock with a piece of twine and he should be all right until tomorrow. I will give him an injection of antiserum to prevent lockjaw and you can renew his poultice every twelve hours."

With those instructions John started to pack away all his instruments, when David interrupted him. "Could you call up in the morning and have a look at my mare? My brother left her back with me and he tells me that she has not been too well in the last few days. She is doing a lot of coughing and has lost a considerable amount of weight"

"Certainly, replied John, "It will give me a chance to drop in and see Prince in the morning as well."

As it was half term, I was staying with my grandparents and soon after breakfast I went into John's house to see if I could help.

"There's not much to do in the surgery," John said, "You've been working so hard that the shelves are full up with bottles and drenches. I am going off in a few minutes to see David McFeeter's mare and we could call in and see how Prince is getting on. I think that they were quite impressed by the purple smoke. Not only is it effective but it is also part of the art of veterinary medicine. I'll meet you in your Uncle Graham's garage in a few minutes."

Full of excitement I rushed back into the house and collected my boots and then went into the garage where John was filling the Popular with petrol. It was always enjoyable to go out with him as he would tell me little stories about many of the farms we passed. I always looked forward to visiting Macosquin to see 'Clinta', the farm where my grandfather was born and I wondered how anyone could have had 13 children in such a small house.

After passing Moneycarry schoolhouse we stopped outside Rob McNulty's smallholding and called in to check on Prince. There was nobody at home but we were pleased to see him bearing full weight on the infected foot and much of the swelling had gone down.

Chapter Twelve

WE DROVE DOWN the road for half a mile then turned up the track to David McFeeter's farm. The house itself was two storeys high, solid, and stone built with a wooden porch at the back door and walls smothered with ivy, giving it a warm, comfortable lived in look. The entrance was stone paved like the kitchen floor and Mrs McFeeter was on her knees inside with scrubbing brush and bucket.

"Hello," she said, "you must be Mr Morrow. I'm Annie McFeeter. David will be back in a couple of minutes. He has just gone up the lane to let the cows out. I'm having to scrub out the kitchen as one of the drains blocked last night and flooded the whole place. Would you like me to give David a shout? But if you want to see Mary, the mare, she is in yon' double door tied up in her stall. She's not very well and has an awful cold.

Thanking her, we walked across the yard and into the stable. Mary was a lovely grey hunter, about 16.5 hands in height with a deep neck and chest. Under normal conditions she looked very handsome with a "hogged" mane and docked tail.

Before entering the building we could her rasping breathing and, as we stood behind her, we could see her great rib cage laboriously heaving in and out. Her ears were down and there was a nasty yellowish discharge from the nostrils and saliva dribbling from her mouth.

John walked up beside her and gently felt along her head and neck. Taking out his thermometer he checked her rectal temperature, listened to her chest with his stethoscope and monitored her pulse at the elbow. At this stage of the proceedings he always pushed his hat to the back of his head which indicated that he was concentrating deeply.

At that moment the door swung open as David arrived in. "Och, hello," he commenced,

"Am I glad to see you. She has got a lot worse since yesterday, she can hardly breathe and the flesh has dropped away from her. Sorry I wasn't here to meet you but I spent a few minutes looking at a heifer that should be calving tonight. What's her problem. Has she got pneumonia?"

"Well, it's like this," said John, "She's a very sick mare. Temperature 105 degrees and she's got strangles quite severely. Her lungs don't sound too bad but the main problem is the swollen glands on the neck. The glands between the jaws and at the back of the jaws are very swollen and pressing in on the throat.

On top of that I reckon that the glands at the back of the throat are also enlarged. All told they have narrowed down the air passage to about a quarter of its normal size. She can't swallow, finds it difficult to cough and is very distressed. This is why it's called strangles!"

"We've got a problem," he continued, "If I treat her as I would a normal strangles, exertion of moving might be too much for her.

On the other hand, if I can lance the glands and drain some of the pus away, it will relieve the pressure on her throat. That is, if she doesn't get too excited."

Anticipating the reply, he said, "Can you get me a pail of hot water, soap and disinfectant, please?"

"You go ahead," replied David, "Treat her as you think best. She could die either way and she's been too good a friend to leave her to suffer."

David fetched the water whilst John went out to the car to collect his instruments and returned in a couple of minutes with a case and a jumble of metal work and leather straps. "Turn her round to face us, David. Quietly, now."

John had a good look at the swellings around the head, prodding them here and there. I do believe that the abscesses are coming to a head, almost at bursting point. I shall have a look at those in the back of the throat. Give me a hand here, Noel. That jumble over there is a Haussman Gag and those straps will hold it on her head like a halter"

I handed over the gag and John adjusted it on the mare's head so if he opened it she could not close her mouth

"Now hold this knife," said John, "When I shout, slip that ring, on the back of it, onto my finger so that the blade lies in my palm." He handed me the blade and ring to hold and turned his attention to Mary. Swiftly opening her jaw with the gag he pushed his hand down her throat momentarily, said "Knife" and I slipped it over the index finger of his right hand. Before Mary had time to complain, his hand was into her mouth for what seemed an instant and was just as rapidly withdrawn.

Mary coughed, John's arm was covered with blood and pus, but instantly her breathing was easier. "There you are old girl, if you don't bleed to death you will probably live. I have lanced both of the pharyngeal glands. Where's that pail of soap and water so that I can get rid of some of this mess."

Ablutions having been completed John gave her another examination, decided that the sublingual glands between the jawbones were "ripe" and carefully, using a lancet, opened up the abscesses. They were both left to drain and David was instructed to disinfect the stables well and keep any other horse away.

By this time Mary was feeling much more relaxed and comfortable so David left her a pail of clean water to clear out her throat. "Thanks very much John. I was very concerned that we would never follow the hounds together again and I'm sure that Mary is even more grateful".

"She's not out of the wood yet, David. Call in the surgery in the morning and I shall give you some powders to give her which will kill the infection. In the next few weeks you should keep a close eye on her in case she develops 'bastard' strangles when other glands throughout the lungs, abdomen and body may abscess and burst. That could be fatal."

As we drove away John looked at me with a twinkle in his eye and said, "you're enjoying seeing practice aren't you Noel. You are becoming quite useful helping with the dispensing in the surgery. Do you think that you would like to be a vet."

"I do indeed," was my reply, "I think that I would like to go to The Royal Dick College in Edinburgh like you and your father. I've got to be a bit careful at the moment though as Gran thinks that animals should not be sick on the Sabbath and that her grandson certainly shouldn't be working on a Sunday." At this stage there was still a lot of hero worship and romance about Edinburgh as Jack Morrow had won quite a few medals as a student.

"Right, you've not finished work yet. There is still a job to do on the way home. We must call in to see Dessie Bell as he has quite a few lame sheep and he wants to get them right before the breeding season." Desmond Bell had spent several years farming in New Zealand before returning home to join the family shipping firm. Most of his week was dedicated to the family business although his great joy was to spend any spare time at home on the farm tending his sheep and black Angus cattle. As he was an extremely competent farmer John did not see him too often.

The farm, covering some 150 acres ran down to the banks of the River Bann near its junction with the Agivey river. The family home was a large Georgian house with bay windows, perched on a promontory, overlooking the river. The view from the front terrace was breathtaking on a sunny morning with the pasture sweeping down to the broad silver ribbon of the Bann, across the rich farming land around Ballymoney and towards the summits of Knocklayd and Croaghan, silhouetted in the distance.

Like so many houses of that era its stark simplicity fitted into the landscape with its backdrop of trees leading up to the road.

As we drove up the avenue and turned off towards the farm buildings we watched a pair of border collies working a batch of Suffolk sheep towards the sheep pens in the corner of the field, each dog taking its own side of the group and immediately responding to the sharp whistled commands. Intent on the job in hand, darting here and there to return a straggler to the flock, now lying, now crawling, but always completely single-minded, as the sheep moved steadily towards the open gate of the sheep pen.

"Aren't they a treat to watch?" said John, "That's Dessie with the crook, working the dogs. He's so well known at the local sheep dog trials for his piercing whistle that he's referred to hereabouts as " Decibel".

By the time that we drew into the yard the lame ewes were being separated out into a small handling pen.

Dessie Bell was a well-built man, in his early forties, with wavy blonde hair just starting to recede from his forehead. He had the florid complexion of a man accustomed to the open-air and pale blue eyes suggestive of Norse blood somewhere in the family line. He treated life very seriously although on occasion, particularly where his family were concerned, would cast away his problems and become full of laughter and fun.

Dressed in an open-necked grey shirt, Fair Isle pullover and a well-worn pair of corduroys he was in his element when handling sheep. He carried over his business efficiency into his farming and kept his standards high. He was known to be a hard taskmaster but had earned the respect of his staff by leading from the front and never expected them to do a job to which he would not turn his hand.

Ditches were cleared and hedges well laid to make them stock proof. The yard itself was neat and tidy with lime-washed buildings contrasting with the glossy black doors and window frames. All the machinery was well maintained and lined up under cover from the elements. Pride of place was occupied by a Ferguson tractor which was very much a working status symbol in the area.

"I must apologise for the state of these feet," said Dessie, "They've been away at pasture for several months and the man in charge has neglected them rather badly. I blame myself as I should have dropped in to see them."

His foreman took hold of a young ewe as we entered the pen and sat her up on her end. The feet were over grown and split. One of the toes on the right fore foot was swollen and had a bloody serum oozing from it.

"What a mess," retorted John," These poor devils must be in a lot of pain. I'll just collect my gear and we can sort out the problem."

"Now, look at this foot. The toes are too long and the wall of the foot has rolled over underneath, trapping a lot of dirt." He picked up his foot shears and knife and rapidly cut away all the overgrown horn until he had the toe back into shape, exposing a raw mass of infected proud flesh.

"Now look at this, Noel. The body has tried to heal the infected wound underneath but it can't heal in the presence of infection and the swelling won't let the infection drain away. I'm going to cut away most of the proud flesh and then dress it with bluestone paste to burn away the rest and give good drainage. Fetch me the bluestone, bandages and cotton wool from the car."

As I scurried away to collect the dressings from the car he finished trimming the foot. After spreading the paste on the cotton wool he placed it on the wound and bandaged it on firmly. There were six more sheep to treat and before leaving we left Dessie feeling much happier, with instructions to remove the dressings in 48 hours. Not only was he happy but I was beginning to realise what life was about.

Chapter Thirteen

SOME WEEKS LATER the house master called me to his study during the morning. "Better spruce yourself up Stuart. You have to report to 'The Chief's' office at 2pm. Don't be late"

The rest of the morning was a purgatory of doubt. I played with my lunch. My mind was a mass of contradictions concerning my reason for this appearance. With shoes freshly polished, nails and face scrubbed and hair slicked back (matron had already straightened my tie.) Not my usual scruffy self I set off on my fateful journey.

Quietly I tapped at the door, knees trembling. The secretary, Nancy Kane, answered my tentative knock and, with knees still trembling, I was ushered into the inner sanctum where 'the Chief' sat at his desk. "Sit down Noel," he said in a brusque but kindly manner. "Thank you Sir!" I managed to mutter.

I sat there firm in the belief that I had besmirched the family name and that expulsion was imminent, or at least the cat o'nine tails.

"Now tell me Noel. You have been here for a year now. Are you enjoying being at Inst?"

"Yes thank you sir!"

"You have improved very much during this year, Noel. Soon you will have to be making your choice for Junior Certificate Examinations. Have you any idea what you want to do in life?"

"Yes sir. I have decided that I would like to be a Vetinary Surgeon" (I couldn't even spell the word at that stage!).

'The Chief' looked at me in amazement, as if I had said a rude word. He expostulated, "What kind of a profession do you call that? Do you know anything about being a vet?"

"Oh yes sir" I replied with the confidence of a student with three months experience under his belt. "I have been going out with Mr Morrow for the past few months and I think that it's great."

At this point the Chief shook his head in sorrow and disbelief. "I know your grandparents very well and I respect them as outstanding people in the town. What do they have to say?

"Well, Dando, that's my grandfather, thinks that it is a good idea."

"And what does your grandmother have to say on the subject, Noel," continued 'the Chief' with a slight smile on his face.

"She thought that it was rather nice to be a professional gentleman sir, but she doesn't really think that I should be working on the Sabbath, 'cos even the servants don't have to work as hard on the Lord's Day!"

A mixture of emotions passed across his face as he tried to maintain his dignity. He knew my grandmother to be a charming old lady with a very religious turn of mind. After a slight pause to collect his thoughts, he continued. "Well Noel, your father is a very well thought of doctor and your brother is studying medicine. Would you like to become a doctor or join your grandfather in his very successful business ?

"The only vets I have known have been dirty old men! Have you talked to your parents. Why don't you try to be a doctor like your father? Think about it and let me know"

"Oh! No sir. I love the country and am determined to be a vet like Mr Morrow in the town."

I escaped from the study in absolute confusion. Would I really end up as a dirty old man? Certainly, Jack and John Morrow were quite tidy. They wore tweed jackets and porkpie hats which looked very respectable in the market.

Beneath the mathematic classroom was the history classroom overseen by 'Baldy' Edwards. He was a nice enough man in himself and quite exact. It was rumoured that he played cricket for Yorkshire. This subject was great if you were interested, but I found that the continuous politicking and enacting new laws to be extremely boring for a budding young vet.

At this time we had a new intake of pupils and during one history lesson there was a 'huck and a cack' on the back row and the sound of spitting. 'Baldy' who was facing the blackboard went all rigid, turned about, "Who made that spitting noise?"

There was a breathless hush as we all waited in anticipation-Then new boy Wullie spoke up. "It was me Sir! I spat on the floor"

"What a disgusting thing to do boy. I hope that it never occurs again."

The sheepish response came back. "I'm sorry Sir. I won't do it again"

"In that case we shall proceed with the South Sea Bubble."

Ten minutes later there was a repeat performance and 'Baldy' turned round slowly, stared, "Was that you again Wullie?"

Honest to the end Wullie said, "Yes Sir. I spat on the wall this time."

The resulting atmosphere was not conducive to learning so we terminated the South Sea Bubble early.

One teacher always stands out above others. In my case it was Vin Smith, freshly returned from the army. Hooray ! – no more Whip Cordner! Vin was blonde with piercing blue eyes which looked through you and an unsmiling mouth. Many boys were very frightened by his approach. He was positive but carried you with him in enthusiasm. We delved deeply into parsing, which I still don't understand.

He taught us the sheer joy of Shakespeare; my love of poetry was revitalised and I even broke through the boundaries of verbal painting by winning a few 'A's for essay writing. After setting alight my love of language his premature death was one of my early periods of mourning when he drowned at Portrush. Now, when writing my books, I work on the premise: never let the truth get in the way of a good story!

When we first arrived at Inst. there were two rugby pitches and all teams had to change in the school and trot over the Ballycairn Road and across a couple of fields to the pitches. This all changed in my last years when the bulldozers moved in and improved the situation, giving us five playing fields and a changing pavilion.

During all these alterations those boarding pupils who were not playing rugby on Wednesday or Saturday mornings were detailed to pick stones from the newly constructed surfaces. We spent many hours, in Wellington boots, stone picking in pretty miserable weather but it kept us occupied.

My great joy was to edge towards the side of the field where there was a six foot drop. Once over the top we were out of sight and would head for the banks of the River Bann. The shallows on the riverside were muddy and lined with rushes which stood well over our heads. This was a magical place inhabited by water birds of all description.

Creeping through the rushes we could see swans, ducks and moorhens and even found several nests. Fortunately, none of the nests were in use at the time as a confrontation with a swan with cygnets could well have been our undoing. Trying to escape when your feet are trapped in oozing mud is not easy.

Nineteen forty five was a memorable year when we celebrated V E Day. We had been listening intently to the news on our cat's whisker radios as the allies closed in on Berlin. When it was eventually announced that the war was over we were all called into room three to listen to 'the Chief'. The room was buzzing with excitement as 'the Chief' entered, followed by the teaching staff. He announced that we were to be given a week off school but must keep up preparations for our exams in June.

At once Basil McCrea suggested that I went home with him to Ramelton in Donegal for a week. As we rushed out into Sausage Park to celebrate, we found Sergeant Vincent issuing all the boarders with thunder flashes and smoke bombs from the army cadet stores. Already the school was engulfed in smoke as Basil and I grabbed our share of the loot and headed back for the 'Gods'. By lunchtime we had bags packed and hurried off to the railway station through the celebrating crowds to catch the train for Derry.

En route to Derry we passed through Limavady. On the platform was a seventeen-stone porter. He was very surprised to hear a thunder flash explode behind him as our train drew away. The next call of interest was when the line ran alongside Eglinton Navy airfield where we left a smoke bomb beside the runway as a keepsake.

As we drew into Derry we had to struggle through the crowds to reach the Lough Swilly bus. I can still remember the printed notice asking passengers not to spit on the floor. We had agreed not to declare our contraband at the customs into Eire. Fortunately nobody was interested in us and we breathed a sigh of relief. Eventually we arrived in Ramelton, unloaded our bags and were welcomed with an ample meal by Basil's mother.

The next few days flew by as we roamed around the town, went for a few cycle rides and I was introduced to his pet trout which lived in their well. We wandered along the banks of the River Lennon, which flows through the town. The river was fairly low and we could walk along the banks and on to an island in the river.

This was a good place to explore for a couple of boys and we quickly formulated a plan of action. We returned to the island half an hour later, checked to see that there was no one in sight and set off the remaining smoke bomb before fleeing back into the house undetected. I understand that it did not take long for the fire service and local gardai to appear. How did an island go up on fire? Nobody knew!

One of my lasting impressions of Ulster, at that time, was the religious divide. I had been brought up with a great sense of fairness and acceptance of other people in society. I was completely bewildered by the dominance of Orangeism and the denigration of the Catholics. This was not about Christianity as we all prayed to the same god. Apart from one very tolerant Catholic boy all the pupils were Protestant. I did not come into contact with any Catholics amongst my peers until I went to Queen's University.

When several of my friends told me that they could know a Catholic just by looking at him I was even more confused as I did not possess this magic insight. I later decided that it was because the Catholics were poorer and less well dressed. I was told not to enter Killowen, the poorer part of Coleraine lest I might be set upon.

On a weekend pass from school I would stay with my grandparents in Hannover Place and I mentioned my worries to my Aunt,

Adden. "Yes!" She said. "Jimmy and I have had to live with this problem but it is changing and people are becoming more tolerant. Your grandfather's parents were brought up in this very bigoted atmosphere. When he went into business on his own he found that half of his customers were Catholic. Being a very even handed man he was increasingly concerned about the situation. To salve his conscience and treat his clients equally he left the Orange order and never attended the Presbyterian Church again. This was a very brave act in the 1920's" The curious situation about the Irish conquest by William of Orange, which Gran did not know, was that he was financed by the Pope.

Many scientists, by their intellect and training find a belief in God difficult to cope with. They are educated to be sceptical and ask questions! How does God satisfy the criteria of a double blind trial?

My antecedents, living in Ulster, during and before the nineteenth century had much less problem with belief. They accepted the garden of Eden, Immaculate Conception and re-incarnation as factual whilst those who delved deeply into theology realised that stories repeated over the centuries became embellished and blurred around the edges. Despite the aims of love and peace enthroned in many faiths the interpretation put upon it by mankind has been the source of many wars across the centuries.

Chapter Fourteen

MY SCHOOL LEAVING results were satisfactory but not enough to enter veterinary college. I resolved to try for the senior certificate in the Isle of Man. This would be great as it would only involve three subjects instead of the seven I was studying in Ireland. The best laid plans....! I quickly found out that senior certificate was much advanced on my school leaving standards, and I was for the first time distracted by working alongside pretty girls.

Back to the Inst. as a day boy was the arrangement and I stayed with my grandparents. I settled in very well and Adden used to teach me to drive a car as I took her to Portrush to play poker every Saturday night. My studies went well and I qualified to enter veterinary college. This year Derek was absent as he had been accepted at Sandhurst as an officer cadet. I never understood how such a gentle person should be interested in warfare.

In that winter of 1947 when temperatures plummeted and the River Bann froze over enough to allow small cars to drive on its icy surface. It also snowed quite deeply and we made use of the Oceana toboggan built by a busy father. It would carry six riders and had independent steering which made it so efficient that we could ride from Carthall, near the school and finish up in Coleraine Diamond over a mile away.

My whole year had been occupied in making applications to veterinary colleges but the earliest vacancies were in four years, particularly if I wanted to attend Ballsbridge College in Dublin and Edinburgh was only taking ex-servicemen. Instead I registered for the agriculture course at Queens University in Belfast in the hope of getting an extra degree.

I left Inst. as a troubled young man, upset by the religious troubles and concerns of being a teenager. I was an avid fan of Maurice

Walsh, an Irish writer, who as a nationalist romanticised the struggle of his countrymen against the English occupation of his beautiful land and particularly against the Black and Tans, who represented the worst of the occupying forces.

I had seen the behaviour of the northern Protestants against the Catholic population in Northern Ireland, which did not impress me, and my sympathies lay with the nationalists at that time.

My first digs were in Botanic Gardens, Belfast run by Tom and Tilly Lynch. There were seven students four Protestant, two Catholic and a communist, which led to interesting discussions. One of these was Noel King who particularly interested me as he had been educated in a turf school. Each pupil attending these schools had to take a block of turf (peat) to provide fuel for warmth and cooking at the school.

The house in Botanic Gardens was rickety, very cold and full of surprises as the banisters kept falling out. I kept one broken banister stuffed up the chimney in case of emergency. Eventually one of the legs of my bed went through a rotten floorboard, which Tom eventually repaired.

The room was so cold when I tried to study in it that action was required. I fixed a double socket in my light. The second socket led to an electric ring on the floor. I would sit on the edge of my bed studying at a card table in the evening. This was a good source of warmth and as I had a saucepan filled with water on top of it I could make tea and boil eggs for supper. I'm sure that mother would have admired my ingenuity if she had only known!

The problem was that Tom kept apologising to me that the fuse box kept blowing, which was quite strange as the electric ring probably required fifteen amps.

The other problem was 'Toby' the beloved, smelly, fat and obnoxious terrier belonging to Tom and Tilly. He was the centre of our hate as he used to attack our trousers on sight. I know that the other lodgers planned his demise, particularly the pharmacy students, and each night at supper time he used to be fed cup cakes loaded with mustard and all things noxious, but he thrived in spite of us.

After three months I decided that I must move up to the new hostel run by Rev Ray Davey, who went on to found the Corrymeela Trust. This was completely different situation, a home from home where one was cared for and joined in the local youth club activities. I even took pleasure in doing the washing up with a pretty girl called Joy Glasgow.

I was very sensitive to the fact that my parents were paying for my university expenses and I spent five shillings a week on myself – five Woodbines, half a pint at the club bar, two games of snooker, and ballroom dancing lessons with Joy at John Dossors Ballroom. In a good week we also had a wild night at the university hop.

To calm my deep worries I went to catholic conversion services at Clonard Cathedral. I gave this up after two services. I had watched the clergy whirling a brass censer, pouring smoke, around his head. I was seriously concerned on a health and safety basis that it might break and kill me so abandoned all hopes of becoming a devout Catholic. Perhaps my own personal belief in a God who was always with me suited so much better.

Chapter Fifteen

MY YEAR AS AN agriculture student was not outstanding as I was called up for national service as soon as I returned to the Isle of Man. I applied to join the Royal Army Veterinary Corps, in the hope that I could work with horses. They accepted me despite my tubercular adhesions and the fact that I was a sympathizer of the IRA at the time.

My basic training was with the Cheshire Regiment at Whittington barracks, Lichfield. These barracks were condemned when my Uncle Bert had trained there in 1914. I didn't take kindly to their unthinking discipline, which appeared illogical to me, but had also made the British army a very efficient force. My only outstanding achievements were on the assault course where I nearly vomited when I had to drive a bayonet into a sack stuffed with straw and the following week on the rifle range when I did not hear the command to cease fire with a Bren gun and nearly shot the sergeant. Would the court martial verdict have been 'homicide' or 'jolly careless'?

After ten weeks I was deemed to be sufficiently trained to be sent to a unit. I was despatched to the Royal Army Veterinary Corps in Melton Mowbray, hoping to end up on the horse lines.

My arrival in Melton Mowbray was an eye opener as I had to wear service dress and a peaked cap, with puttees. The major problem was that the Corps did not have a cap large enough, so I had to wear a beret for six weeks whilst they constructed a cap of the correct dimensions.

As requested I was allocated to the horse lines, which was already occupied by stable lads and jockeys, so I was very much the amateur when it came to riding out.

A new face that sounds educated must be tested out, so I was ordered by the lance corporal in charge to clean out the stable drains by hand. I had no problems hand shovelling horse dung which I had done many times before, so I was warily accepted. We had a large and irascible Hanoverian mare in the horse lines and Derek, a small jockey lad, must have offended her sensitivities, so she promptly bit him in the rump and flung him out over the top of the half door.

Of course all the soldiers in the horse lines had to do their stint of duty, keeping an eye on the horses at night and feeding when required. When we had talked to all the horses and the night grown longer, it was possible to have a quick snooze in a stable once the duty officer had done his tour of duty.

Any empty loose-boxes were used to house sick army dogs. The unit trained dogs of all capabilities, guard, tracking and mine-detection. When the guard dogs occupied a loose-box only the brave entered inside alone as they were trained to attack and respond to a series of commands from their handler. During a weekend guard duty it could become quite boring as there was little to do. Guard dogs in the loose boxes were fed regularly and eventually developed a rapport with their feeders so we could go into the box with them. They automatically reacted to commands and would respond to 'Lie'. The dog would lie as two of us would sit in diagonal corners.

I would call 'Zane' the dog and command him to lie at my feet. Next command was 'sit'. I would then point to my friend, Wilf, in the opposite corner and shout 'watch' followed by 'attack', at which point the confused dog would launch himself across the box at Wilf. A sharp 'sit' then 'lie' from Wilf would have Zane lie obediently, followed by a reversal when I would be attacked. This game helped to fill in the hours on a Sunday afternoon.

I had a short spell of leave and returned home, elegant in my smart uniform. Brother Derek was also finishing his leave so we spent a few days together whilst he regaled me with tales of his exploits with the colonel's daughter.

My sister Jane had arrived from university with a boyfriend. She appeared to be a bit moonstruck as girls do in these situations and asked me if I knew of Mona Brew, a wise woman, who told fortunes. She also owned a mule! I replied that I knew her cottage in the North of the Island and would take her there.

When we found the cottage we were invited inside. "Meet my little Timmy" she said looking into a birdcage with an odd coloured canary. "He's a mule. That's a canary crossed with a finch."

We sat down and Jane crossed her palm with the customary silver. Mona took her hand and examined the palm carefully. After a few minutes she put it down and quietly said. "This is very interesting dear. I can see you getting married next year but not to this gentleman who is with you," indicating her boy friend. "Before this takes place your family will suffer a great disaster about which I cannot tell you." We thanked her profusely, very confused about the message.

It came to pass that she did find a new boyfriend and fixed the wedding day for the 25th July without any sign of problems.

Back at Melton Mowbray I was called up to the quartermaster's office one day and was informed that I as I had been educated I was to be promoted to despatch clerk. Not realising the 'honour'. I was told to report to the office next morning at 8.00 am. On time I reported to the office sergeant (a writer of awful poetry).

"You will sit at this desk here," he said, indicating a long desk, stuck in a corner, with a pretty view of a green and buff wall. "Each morning at 8.30 sharp you will receive all the out-going mail. In this 'ere ledger you will enter the source, our reference and destination of each piece of mail (with the time) and return them to my desk for despatch."

"Certainly, sergeant. I shall do my utmost to keep up with the office procedure."

Now, office work has never been my favourite occupation, but I decided to give it all my efforts. I might even attain promotion. After receiving the post and cataloguing the record I found that I was finished by 9.45. I realised that this was a slack day and, after delivering my mail, resorted to busying myself looking at the MoD green wall. Shortly afterwards I was sent to the guard room with the mail to be posted.

Soon after lunch I returned to the green wall, examined it carefully and resorted to composing poetry and doodling. The next thing that I knew was that the Sergeant was looking over my shoulder. "What's this then?" "Er, sorry sergeant, but I was at a loose end. Is it possible to read a book during slack periods?"

"No, it's bloody not. You can see some of my poetry and then look at the wall." He then slapped a few papers in front of me with his 'pomes' which nowadays would be regarded as pornographic literature.

After work I was walking across the parade ground with David Ball, also a budding veterinary student. Marching towards us we saw Farrier Sergeant Major McLeod. We came to attention and saluted smartly. We were not used to being addressed by an officer of such rank. "Ball," he commenced. "I know that you want to be a vet. Where do you come from?"

"London sir!"

"Bloody big place. Whereabouts in London?"

Looking straight ahead, as you do in these situations, David replied, "Wandsworth Sir"

"Ha Ha! Next thing is you will tell me it's Wandsworth prison!"

"Yes, it is sir!"

"Damned cheek and insolence. Consider yourself on a charge!"

"No sir! I'm sorry but my father is padre in the prison sir!"

"The two of you could spend some time polishing your buttons! You are dismissed."

It occurred to me that if I had made mistakes in the office I might have been returned to the horse lines. However, I was on the way up the ladder. Instead I was sent off to a course in Anstey to train as a Part Two orders clerk. Now this was reward indeed – no extra money above my 18 shillings a week.

When I returned fully trained I was allowed to sit by the sergeant, who kept slipping me his porny poems. Each day I would receive orders from the adjutant's office, which I would type onto the daily orders sheet. I had never used a typewriter so I slogged away all day trying to attain perfection. The orders were then printed out and despatched to the various offices and messes by the cycle orderly of the day. This was constructive work although quite boring. Not quite the thing for a vet! I was rapidly learning what I didn't want to do in life!

Working in the office meant that my guard duty nights were spent as cycle orderly, delivering Part Two orders and spending the night operating the camp telephone exchange and redirecting calls. Most of the calls were for the officers mess, some from young Guards officers wanting to visit and spend the weekend with the Quorn Hunt. Some were polite, others incredibly rude and arrogant to me, a humble soldier.

One advantage of being telephone orderly was that I could listen in to poker games being played at the exchange and chat up the telephonists.

All went well until somebody in the Sergeants mess complained that I had not delivered Part Two Orders, which made him miss an appointment. It did occur to me that this might be an invention to cover up his own failings but rank counts. Next morning I was marched in under guard before the adjutant and accused of behaviour prejudicial to military order and good discipline.

Despite my protestations I was assigned to do 'jankers' for a week. What a lark being the latrine wallah for seven days. Not a care in the world with almost no responsibilities except looking busy when your betters looked in.

One of the assets of being away from home was to learn to get drunk like a gentleman in our local, The Welby Inn, where we enjoyed

Barley wine which was moderately lethal. We could not over imbibe as the hill back to the camp was very steep. The only exception was a little jockey lad who regularly returned in the early hours, tripping over beds and singing loudly, much to the annoyance of the rest of the barrack room, so we adopted the technique of gently tipping him out of the window so that he could sleep it off in the onion bed!

On the whole we were not a highly efficient fighting force in Melton Mowbray. I can only recall one drill session and when Brigadier Heveningham came to inspect this fine body of fighting men we had forgotten how to present arms. A bit like Slattery's Light Dragoons!

During our time off in the evenings we would wander across the fields and inspect the pig farm and on our return after dark we would ride the colonel's horse bareback across the paddock.

It was during a warm summer afternoon on the first of July that I was summoned to the adjutant's office to hear the news that my brother Derek had been killed in Germany. Completely stunned, I wandered across the pasture and wept for hours. Early next morning I was sent home on compassionate leave to find my parents were inconsolable.

Indeed, my mother, who was diabetic, was having daily crises with the condition and I was very sad to depart at the end of my leave. After several weeks of disasters with my mother's diabetes the RAVC granted me a compassionate discharge.

I was not very concerned as I could not appreciate the benefits of national service when I was absorbed in pursuing a veterinary career. It was at this juncture that I recalled Mona Brew's prediction and Jane was due to marry soon.

It was a very tragic time when we received Derek's effects and his ashes from his unit in Germany. We had made previous arrangements and had his ashes scattered in Port Erin Bay as a family group. He and I had grown up together in the town and sixty years later I still find the memory very poignant.

It was just as well that I had a year at home before entering veterinary college. I could act as a buffer between my mother and concerned people who wished to see her. Dad had the solace of being busy at work but she remained at home with her thoughts and was resorting more than normal to the gin bottle.

Later in the year I had been horse riding with the vet's daughter, Irene, after which we had to clean out stables, feed and groom. I arrived back home in the evening to meet a young lady who my mother introduced as Margaret Walker, a friend of Derek's, who was teaching at the Girl's High School. She was very pretty, dressed in a well cut grey suit, with curved collars and a bright intelligent face. When she stood up I could see that she had a waistline which I could have spanned with my hands. She was such a slim creature that she would break in a strong wind.

Definitely not my type, like the outdoor horsey girls who didn't mind getting mucky.

I was so engrossed in making my estimate of this young lady that it didn't occur to me that I too was under scrutiny. Margaret was quite surprised that this was the brother of the charming young officer she had met previously. He wore a tatty old jersey, covered with hay, his hair was every-which-way and he seemed to smell very strongly of horses! After he changed his clothes, at his mother's request, he reappeared looking fairly presentable and definitely smelling more wholesome!

Following a bite of supper I offered to walk Margaret home as I was curious to meet yet another of Derek's conquests. They had met on the Isle of Man boat when she was returning to Liverpool after her job interview as a P.E teacher at the Girl's High School and he had suggested that she called to see mum if she felt lonely.

Since Derek's death the remit had changed and she was giving mum companionship. We chatted away quite happily until I left her at her lodgings. I told her one day about the mysterious gift possessed by a farmer's wife. She had the ability to stop an animal bleeding. This was a bit magical. Not only that but I heard on the grapevine that she was banned from the slaughter house because of this ability.

Margaret capped this tale with a story of a girl at High School. Part of her physical education duties were to inspect pupils feet regularly for the presence of verrucas. One girl had a very large verruca and she suggested that she consulted a doctor. After a pause the girl said that she had visited a wise woman to have it charmed off. Within four days the problem had vanished! This evidence of the occult set us both wondering. We had been brought up to believe that 'occult' was black magic. The dictionary explanation was that it meant 'unknown' or 'unseen' but not evil.

During the following year I spent many hours working in the veterinary practice and exercising the horses. I even learnt to dismount over the head! We went to horse shows and many gymkhanas. Often when I returned home I would find Margaret visiting. We would be sent off to make supper together and developed a strong affection for one another. I would take her off to all my childhood haunts and many times watched the sunset over Peel or Port Erin.

Realising that our feelings for one another were deepening, Margaret decided that she must leave the island as I had five years college studies ahead and she did not wish to affect my veterinary studies in Dublin. After much hesitation she arranged to go to Pietermaritzburg in South Africa as a physical education instructor at a girl's school.

Parting is such sweet sorrow and we both decided to go our separate ways until her return to England in four years time. She departed for Capetown in the summer and I prepared to go to Veterinary College in Dublin during September.

Chapter Sixteen

For I have learned

To look on nature,not as in the hour

Of thoughtless youth;but hearing oftentimes

The still, sad music of humanity,

Nor harsh nor grating,though of ample power

To chasten and subdue. And I have felt

A prescence that disturbs me with the joy

Of elevated thoughts; a sense sublime

Of something far more deeply interfused,

Whose dwelling is the light of setting suns,

And the round ocean and the living air,

And the blue sky, and in the mind of man:

A motion and a spirit which impels

All thinking things, all objects of all thought,

And rolls through all things.

Lines composed a few miles above Tintern Abbey1798-
William Wordsworth

IT HAD BEEN A warm summer when young men have the urge to entertain fair maidens and we had lots of fun together. Indeed at the following New Year I heard on the grapevine that I was reported to be engaged to seven different girls and even married to one lucky lady. This was the Manx gossip line working at speed.

There was very little basis for the stories, but it boosted my ego tremendously to be regarded as the 'in' man, even if I was footloose and fancy free-with no money. Oh for a girl with lots of acres!

I went off to Milford in Donegal with the folks for two weeks of fishing on Lough Fern with Paddy McGettigan as our gillie. It was my kind of country where we had made friends and the girls at the Ceilidhs were as pretty as pictures.

Mum would visit her friend Jean McDowell and dad and I would collect Paddy as we departed for the day. The lake was shallow and we always managed to bring back a dozen fish for the hotel, and sometimes the odd salmon. Possibly the next day we would fish tidal waters for slob trout or even a stretch of the Lennon, searching its murky waters for salmon.

Walking across the heather with our two pointers and Paddy's setter, shooting grouse was always a delight. I would have gone solely to admire the pointers, just to watch them freeze and point their quarry.

It was the kind of town where it would take half an hour to walk a hundred yards up the street because the bookie, the draper, the priest or the Garda sergeant would stop for a bit of craic. You got a lot of things done – slowly. We would return to the hotel for dinner and then into the bar for a few drinks and just listen to the talk. At ten o'clock the barman Pat Finney might usher us into the snug at the back.

"You see gentlemen, little Mickey O'Donohue is in for the evening as he's a bit addicted to the drink. Just after closing time at ten-thirty Sergeant Kelly has told us he is going to make a raid to catch illegal drinkers. It's always the same. In he walks and says 'Mr O'Donohue, you are drinking out of hours and I must arrest you'. At this point he leads your man off to the Garda barracks and fills in the necessary forms for which Mickey will be fined. The hotel pays the fine, Mickey has a free night's drinking and Sergeant Kelly reports back to headquarters that he has curbed after-hours drinking in the town.

The sergeant was a member of the hotel poker school which consisted of the owner, the doctor, the priest and the draper. Together they ran the town peaceably. The only thing that upset the sergeant was an Oxford English accent which reminded him of the Black and Tans during the troubles in the 1920s. I was standing outside the hotel one day when a Sunbeam Alpine coupé drew up beside the sergeant. The driver, an immaculately-coiffured lady was heard to say in a plummy voice "Excuse me OFFICER! Could you tell me the way to Downings?"

Courteous to the end the sergeant replied, "Certainly madam. Just follow your nose down the road for eight miles and you can't go wrong." At this point he turned and walked away minding his own business, but had barely taken four steps when the plummy voice continued, "Oh OFFICER I'm going to stay at the Beach Hotel. Can you tell me if it is near the strand."

His body language spoke out as Sergeant Kelly went all stiff and stick-like. I could almost see the hairs on his neck standing erect. Turning around slowly he stared at the lady "Ah M'am! If I remember correctly, at a full tide you can stand on the verandah and pish into the sea!" Having delivered his message he quietly walked away.

My other memory of Milford was when Billy Hunter, the vet, heard that the local pharmacist was dispensing antibiotics to farmers without any knowledge of the disease.

"Come with me" he said and we drove into town, straight into the chemist's shop where Billy Hunter grabbed the pharmacist by the collar, pulled him half way across the counter and threatened to strangle him if he played fast and loose with his customers' cattle. Problem solved!

It was a good holiday and my last as I had been accepted at college. After it ended the folks left me in my digs, right opposite the Dublin show ground. Before leaving dad gave me his chequebook and said "I hope that you will always spend less than ten pounds a week until you graduate." For that gesture I was eternally grateful. At that we embraced and they headed back home.

The landlady in Dublin was very welcoming and I met my fellow lodger, Jim O'Brien, who was also going to the veterinary college. We went down to the college in Ballsbridge for a scout around and were quite disappointed. As we entered the gates we were presented with a square of brick buildings which appeared to be very unloved and derelict. Through a first floor window two ladies moved around busily which indicated the office and an archway opened through a side building to a row of loose boxes. Out of the boxes several bored horses exhibited weaving movements and two or three men in white coats walked about impressively.

We knocked at the door labelled 'Reception' and were greeted by a secretary who broke off from her typing. "Good afternoon. You will be part of the new intake of students. I have several books of notes which will interest you", she said, picking up three large books for each of us. "Tomorrow morning at nine am. you will be interviewed in the lecture theatre by the principal, Professor T.G Brown who will advise you on textbooks, lectures and clothing."

After a couple of pints to get to know one another we headed back to our digs to unpack our trunks. Jim was also a doctor's son from Sheffield and enjoyed rugby. He was currently training with Landsdowne rugby club and was looking forward to the challenge of our course.

The next morning we arrived early to find the courtyard swarming with students. We arrived in the lecture theatre to find about 30 students of all shapes and sizes sitting on the benches. There were only two girls in our year, one a pretty blonde and the other a brunette with a plait arranged around her head like a halo. I was intrigued to think that these would be my companions for the next few years.

At that moment T.G. Brown, the principal, arrived in the theatre and greeted us as no doubt he did every year. He told us to report to the office where we would receive a list of required textbooks and dissection kits along with white coats which were all available in Grafton Street. He suggested that we all got to know each other and turned up in the morning prepared for anatomy practicals and lectures.

The next morning we arrived at anatomy lectures and then straight into anatomy practicals. Being feisty and immature young men there was much throwing of pieces of liver and bits of carcass at each other. The girls escaped the worst of our attacks. All the cadavers had been injected with formalin to preserve the carcasses. It was very pungent and we continually had to seek fresh air as our eyes were streaming. However we came to no harm and it always amuses me that today we have to handle formalised tissues in vacuum cabinets to avoid its toxicity.

All our carcasses were horses, suspended on their backs from the ceiling so a lot of our time was taken up looking into the abdomens.

To me the fascination of anatomy and physiology was the explanation as to how things actually worked. I was in my element and spent many happy hours poring over my textbooks – I even forgot about being a forensic scientist for seagulls. My fellow students were a pleasure and gently teased me about my Northern Presbyterian roots. "Ah! You're alright even if you do kick with the left foot. We'll test you now and share a pint of porter"

I found exams quite daunting and had a couple of re-sits. I had six years experience behind me when I entered college. I trod the middle path – rugby, fishing, girls (in that order) and enough work to get through my exams. Fortunately these were not the days of CVs, which can deceive and bloat one's self esteem.

One always finds one's level in a community and we soon formed a group. Bert Harris, a gangling Belfast lad was accompanied by his sister, Doreen, the aforementioned blonde. There was Mike Gahan, a handsome Nordic blonde who shared my love of rugby and fishing, and Dick Nunn, who was one of the Anglo-Irish gentry.

One of our fellows was an IRA sympathiser and was later prosecuted for repatriating an Irish painting from the Royal Art Gallery in London back to its native country.

Eventually Bert, Jim O'Brien and I all moved digs to Mount Merrion and travelled into college on our bicycles as it appeared that nearer town they found us to be a bit noisy. There we found that we were further away from the bright city lights and set out rules for studying each night. Work each evening unless we became very bored. Wednesday we worked until nine pm and then headed off to Goatstown pub for a pint.

Saturday meant no work, so it was two pints and then off to a dance to ease our limbs after rugby. Country dances were interesting to say the least. This was a time when young catholic girls were taught of the dangers of men who might compromise a young girl's future.

The cosmopolitan types from overseas and England were like a smoking fuse. I have seen shy country Irish youths, after half an hour of summing up the talent, walk across the floor to where girls were doing the same. Offering his hand he would mutter "Excuse me miss. Would you care to hit the floor a slap?" After a few dances with the same girl he would summon up his courage. "Ah miss! It's been a lovely evening. Are you catered for after the dance?"

Those were the days! We were invited to a party one evening by Angela, a pretty young girl who was educated at the Loretto Convent. It was a friendly evening with a few beers and lots of music and friendly chatter. I was sitting beside her on the settee when somebody turned off the lights whereupon I leaned across and kissed this little charmer. As the lights were turned on again she looked at me in wide eyed amazement. "What did you do that for at all?" I had forgotten her convent upbringing.

Our veterinary studies engulfed our lives completely. No such a thing as free afternoons like the medical or arts students. Bert and I were also working for our concurrent BA degrees at Trinity. Mike and I played rugby three days a week and on occasion I felt the necessity for female company which eased the pressure. Doreen and I developed a firm friendship, which has lasted for 55 years.

Some of the ghosts of my Ulster experiences lived with me and I showed little inclination to attend church. One Sunday morning I was wandering aimlessly in Donnybrook when I came upon a Protestant church and went in to enjoy the quiet of the service. As I went in I saw Doreen sitting in the balcony and went to join her as she was always calm and composed. The sermon was not the fire and brimstone stuff that I had met in Ulster which made me think more deeply about my beliefs, and the fact that I already had a belief in a Greater Being but not in an established church.

As the weather improved Mike and I used to spend weekends away camping and fishing beside a wee cottage at Gara Bridge in Westmeath. We lived like fighting cocks, as the farmer's wife insisted that we had rice pudding brought to us each day lest we faded away. Evening time brought on a thirst for Guinness and we spent many happy evenings enjoying the craic in the local pub.

Each year we had a ball at the Metropole Hotel in O'Connell Street. It was always a good evening and a few times I was able to take Doreen as my partner.

Every fortnight, regular as clockwork, I would receive long newsy letters from Margaret in South Africa, although I was rather remiss in that department. I could only visualise the heat and sights, and I did not think far beyond our situation in Dublin due to the pressure of work.

Each time the professional exams grew near we had a technique of dealing with learning. We would all take a few small index cards in our pockets on which we had written pertinent points on the subject. Whilst we were pondering over a pint of Guinness, out would come a card for interrogating our companions. It seemed to work as we struggled through our exams!

During each holiday I was at home in the Isle of Man seeing practice and becoming more proficient all the time. I was helping with operations on the farm, removing the odd afterbirth under supervision and on one momentous day I was sent off on my own to suture a wound on a sows flank. Students were allowed more freedom to treat animals in Ireland. Indeed some students did locums in their final eighteen months.

When my college career finished I had spent 13 years as an assistant and student, which helped greatly in dealing with clients and handling animals.

One of the advantages of living in Dublin was that dad bought a car, which I could use so that he did not have to hire one when he came over on holiday each year. Often I would join my parents as they would inevitably end up in Milford in County Donegal either on a fishing or shooting holiday.

This was great as I could go and see practice with Billy Hunter in Milford. The practice was very different from the Isle of Man as the farms were much smaller and the owner was out working all day. As a consequence the vet and farmers wife were left in charge to handle the animals, with grandpa giving a hand. Billy and I had a technique where he would walk up beside a cow left at pasture and grab its tail whilst I would make a dive, grab her by the horns and wrestle her into submission, in order to examine her.

Billy did have a case of bracken poisoning on a farm where the cow went mad and tried to charge and kill everyone. Billy stood behind a wall and killed her with an axe as she attacked him.

Quite a few times he would take me to farms where he used his skill as a water dowser in order that they could dig a well for a water supply. He showed his skill using a hazel twig. Not only could he dowse for water but was able to tell the depth of the water source. This was an accomplishment that was completely new to me and I have used it on several occasions since that time. Once more I was involved with the occult!

When we eventually finished our college careers it meant the parting of the ways for many of us, leaving behind the cosseted student life and going to seek a job. We all got through our finals successfully except Mike who had to resit one exam in September.

I was particularly pleased as for the first time I came out top in medicine practicals. I had never visualised being top in anything. Our landlady was overjoyed and left a bottle of Guinness each on the stairs with a note. "You gentlemen must be absolutely full of knowledge."

Many doubts filled our minds concerning our abilities to succeed in practice. With whom? Where? And would we be able to make a success in practice ? Bert was aiming to practice in Ulster, Doreen intended to show-jump her horses all summer. Jim O'Brien had decided that a vet's life was not for him and was changing over to study medicine in Sheffield.

Mum and Dad were coming over to our graduation followed by a fishing holiday and Margaret was also joining them, as she had returned from South Africa. This would probably be the last of our fishing trips. We said our farewells and I arranged to contact Bert and Doreen later in the summer after I had sorted out a job. I had been offered employment in Loughborough, Leicestershire.

Graduation day arrived and I went to the airport early to meet Mum, Dad and Margaret. I hurried out into the arrivals hall and soon spotted dad, fishing rod in hand and mum beside him in a powder blue two piece.

Then Margaret appeared in the doorway, a vision in a figure-enhancing yellow suit, sun-blessed tan, cherry lips and eyes the colour of corn flowers topped by a cheeky red hat poised on her golden hair. I was stunned! This was not the Margaret I had seen off to Africa. She had a poise and self-confidence that completely bowled over the rugged young rugby player who could take or leave the opposite sex. I must have stood open mouthed before rushing across to kiss her. The rest of the day was spent in constant talk and excitement as we wined and dined together.

The next day, after the graduation ceremony, we headed to Corofin in the County Clare. We stayed in a quiet country house where we had lots of time to fill in our five years apart. Each morning during that golden summer we would row round the lake fishing for pike or perhaps a foolish salmon. We caught a few six-pound jack pike which we enjoyed for the evening meal until one morning Margaret landed an eighteen-pound pike – larger than I had ever seen! For the young lover there was no envy, but just joy at her success.

The only other guest at the hotel was a retired Indian civil servant who had two dogs, one an adult retriever and the other a six-month-old pointer pup. He never spoke to them and they would lie at the porch of the hotel whilst he was inside. If the pup tried to slip across the threshold of the door she was pushed outside by the older dog.

I was curious to know why he never called them and why they were so obedient. He told us later that when hunting in India silence was essential and the dogs obeyed hand signals only and hence had no names. When he went into town the dogs followed him to the garage. He placed his cap on the ground and they lay there until his return.

I said to Margaret that I was going to Loughborough for a job interview, and asked if she would come with me whilst she looked around for a job. She was slightly reticent and replied that she had really returned to England to sort out her feelings as she had been going out with another man in South Africa. Alarm bells sounded as I realised that I might lose this lovely nymph who had bewitched me. I agreed not to be too insistent but thought that a couple of weeks together might help us both sort out our future.

After our idyllic holiday we headed for Loughborough and I attended my interview with Hugh Bryson, a fellow Dublin graduate. We both saw eye-to-eye as it was a mainly large animal practice with a growing pet clientele. His only weakness in my opinion was that he had not missed a lecture at college whilst I had regarded compulsory tuition with a more relaxed attitude.

Hugh was the ideal employer for a new graduate and made a point of saying that if ever I had problems, day or night, he would be available to assist. We liked him and I arranged to start work within a month. In the meanwhile Margaret saw several interesting jobs but decided that PE advisor for Lancashire was not her scene.

Eventually a position came up in a comprehensive school in Shepshed near Loughborough, which meant that we could spend a lot of time together. The tender trap was closing on this young bachelor!

Margaret rented a flat in Loughborough and we decided that she could try her growing cookery skills on me each weekend. When we first met she could hardly boil water, whilst I had been making cakes, drop scones and potato bread for lots of years. This fact has been disputed for many years but I still remain confident in my attributes.

We did enjoy that winter, one of the coldest for years. I was constantly having to pick pigeons off the road which were too cold and weak to move. What did impress me was that one of our extensive pig farm clients would turn his pregnant sows into a snowy field with a pile of loose straw. The sows in their turn would have a litter in the straw nest and lie happily in the straw with the little pigs suckling, scampering around or sleeping snuggled up to mum's warm body.

Under Hugh's tutelage I became much more confident in practice. He was without doubt one of the most honest of men. If he called to visit a back yard pig enterprise in a cottage, he would accept a dozen eggs as payment and assiduously enter this transaction into his ledger for tax purposes.

There was a wonderful housekeeper, Florence, who kept the wheels turning. I would receive an early morning call to visit a milk fever case. I had to collect a bottle of calcium borogluconate from her which she had prepared and sterilized before my arrival. This very hot bottle was thrust into my hands with a list of instructions which she had given to the farmer to sit the cow up and place a straw bale behind to support it. She helped to save many a cow's life with her strict instructions. Her magnesium bottles were similar. Concentrated magnesium from which I had to inject fifty ml into the muscle. Lots of these would abscess as the solution was so concentrated but their lives were saved.

Florence's weakness was always evident when she answered the telephone and was seen genuflecting. This told us that it was the local landowner, Lord Belper, where her father had been gardener, who required our attention.

That springtime I was invited back to join the practice in The Isle of Man. Whether it was the season or the thought of separating from Margaret, I proposed to her and amazingly was accepted. We were both in heaven and Margaret contacted the Manx education authority and found that there would be a job vacancy in Douglas later in the year.

This was a great opportunity for us both and as soon as we returned to the island to work with Geoff Stubbs we looked around for somewhere to live and settled for Peel. I could work on the west side and come in to Douglas for surgeries.

This worked very well and we married in Formby the following August. After some months I found that working with Geoff was different to being a student and he started becoming irascible, partly due to his lifestyle. Our personalities were clashing and after two years, when our son Donal had arrived on the scene, we parted by mutual consent. Part of the reason was that I had a yen for far-away places after Margaret's adventures in Africa when she saw a lot of the country.

Our initial thought was to move to New Zealand but in those days when flying was expensive it meant cutting oneself off from one's family. Eventually we arranged to go to Canada on an assisted passage to work for the government for six months. On the face of it this was ideal, as we had a five-day boat journey on the Empress of Britain to Montreal and then a three-day trip to Winnipeg, where I would start carrying out meat inspection in a slaughter house.

Fortunately, I managed to rent an apartment near to Canada Packers slaughterhouse where I was to work. It was an older building and very comfortable. The only drawback was the antiquated heating system with a boiler servicing all apartments. The temperatures inside would approach ninety degrees which meant that we had to put saucepans of water on the radiators to increase the humidity somewhat. The problem was residual static electricity in the room which meant that sparks flew between our noses when we kissed or I received a shock when turning on the light switch!

Turning up for work at six a.m. was a revelation. I had to walk across an enormous car park full of American cars, built like pregnant whales. The place was alive with men in hard hats crowding into the building, which was redbrick and three storeys high.

Eventually I was directed to the veterinary office where I met the chief veterinarian. He was a man of 60 years plus called McLeod, who told me to sit down with a mug of tea whilst I introduced myself. "With your name you should do alright" he commented. "Religion presbyterian. If you vote conservative there is no reason why you should not rise to the top of the service."

I was amazed to hear that Scots and Irish protestants largely emigrated to Canada whilst the United States had many catholics. Lord! Would I never escape from religion?

I was taken into the common room for vets and technicians and introduced as the latest import from the 'old country'. Although many of my fellow workers had originated from over the world, Britain was regarded as the old country. I was supplied with overalls and boots plus a hard hat (extra large) along with a belt which carried meat knives, sharpening steel and meat hook.

These were the tools of my trade. Another vet called Brian took me up to the slaughtering hall and introduced me to the slaughter men. One, Steve Baraniuck, who became a good friend, was of enormous build and offered me his hand, within ten seconds I was on my back so strong was his grip. "Welcome Limey. If you have trouble let me know." As a Ukranian orphan he had been brought up by two old English spinsters who fed him crumpets for tea.

Brian took me up to the slaughter line where the meat inspectors worked and showed me the rudiments of commercial meat inspection. Look to your left. The cattle are driven up a ramp from the ground floor into a yard where they enter one by one into the 'knocking box' where the head is held in a neck tie. Above them a slaughterman stands and hits them on the head with a sledgehammer loaded with a blank cartridge. The animal drops instantly and, before it can recover consciousness has been bled out.

The carcass is then pulled up by the legs to an overhead rail where it moves around the room where it is examined for disease, butchered and eventually leaves the factory to head to the final destination. Our job is to check the animal at all stages for signs of disease and if necessary side-track it for further examination. You will stand here all day, two hours on and two hours off. My heart sank. I joined the profession to treat live animals but the Canadian government had paid my fare so I must stick it out for the statutory six months.

It was not all bad as my fellow workers came from all over the world and I heard many languages spoken. Ex Desert Rats and German Afrika Corps veterans worked shoulder to shoulder. The pay was good and I knew exactly what I had to do. If I picked up diseased tissues I would hand them in to be taken to the laboratory and that was the last I heard of them for two months.

This rather soured my view on working for the government where it was comfortable if one didn't rock the boat. I was very upset on seeing Jewish religious slaughter where a large bull could be suspended by its hindlegs for half an hour until it had its throat severed. Where was my vocation as a healer?

I saw a lot of Margaret and Donal and we could go into town and do our shopping in the snow- Gosh! It was cold with a brilliant blue sky although the temperature was about fifteen degrees below zero.

When the weather eased I decided to take a few driving lessons as my international licence was due to expire. After two lessons my instructor offered me a job as a driving tutor! I did get my licence, but I was also job-hunting as meat inspection was driving me to screaming pitch.

Chapter Seventeen

I HEARD ABOUT A job in Neepawa, a small town in the prairie about a hundred miles west of the city. We drove out one weekend for interview with Bill Brydges for this opportunity to join a large animal practice. We took to each other straight away and Bill told me that they set out each morning at eight o'clock and finished when the calls stopped coming. It was almost entirely beef herds with some horses as they were still used a lot on the farms.

Up to the previous year Bill had driven three hundred horsepower Chryslers until his local garage suggested that he traded them in for Volkwagon Beetles. He laughed until he was shown how well they performed in the winter snows so he now owned five beetles.

They were ideally suited to driving across the prairie, had no water freezing problems and were light enough to drive across snowbound pastures. When it did sink through the snow crust I would leave the engine running and dig out the wheels to give them purchase. It is a bit embarrassing when the car takes off on its own and I had to chase it. One of its great assets was the engine weight over the back driving wheels which meant that we were able to tow large American sedans out of the ditches into which they had slid.

We joined the practice in the springtime, when the snow had cleared. Neepawa was a small town lying in the prairie, surrounded by bush with the main navigation features being the grain silo towers scattered about the country. They were all painted red and had their names painted across the roof, which was a great navigation landmark for planes from the nearby Macdonald airbase.

For me, this was a great adventure, meeting farmers from all nationalities and townships such as Polonia, Ukrainia and Berlin. Ethnic groups had settled in these parts and maintained their own customs and language. It was fairly common to see a black bearded man, dressed in black, walking along the road with his woman staggering along behind carrying a heavy suitcase as befitted her situation in life. These may have been members of the Mennonite or Hutterrite groups who had settled in the province. They were sects with extreme religious views who had fled from Europe to escape persecution.

Much of our work was with groups of animals who had been brought in from the bush for treatment. Several times I was called out to batches of cattle that had broken in to the granary when the farmer was absent. On his return he would find these hapless animals had stuffed themselves with grain and then gone to the trough for a good drink of water. The grain had swelled and started to ferment with the result that the seventy gallon paunch or first stomach had bloated enormously creating pressure on the heart resulting in death.

In one such incident I drove into the cattle yard to see twenty bloated cattle staggering round the yard. We got hold of the first one and a large kitchen knife was thrust into my hand. Time was of the essence. Hygiene and sterilisation came second! Two handed, I drove the knife into the stomach behind the last rib and pulled down to make a nine inch incision. I was the lucky one as the man behind me received the full jet of grain and water in the face. It must have travelled about six feet, so great was the pressure. The steer at once stopped staggering and gasping. Then quickly on to the next four beasts who showed an equally rapid recovery after being stabbed.. This was what I had trained for! We stood back and surveyed the remaining cattle that did not appear to be as severely affected. Some looked sick, a few were off their legs-a pitiful sight!

"Let's grab each one," I said "or we could still lose all of them. Too much protein can kill them so we must get rid of it through the gut."

We held each bullock and I passed a rubber tube down the throat to the stomach. Using a funnel we poured into each animal two pints of liquid paraffin, a pint of linseed oil and a large handful of Nux Vomica powder. The nux vomica contains strychnine which increases bowel movement expelling the toxic grains. It also stimulated the animals which were becoming very depressed. Each one received vitamin B to help cleanse the system.

The final move was to stitch up the wounds in those cows that I had stabbed and try and remove any grain which might have fallen into the abdominal wound. It was a close call but only one animal died.

The same problem can occur when horses get into the feed bin. I was called out to a couple of large Percheron draught horses who had dined unwisely in the feed bin. My problem was administration of liquid. They are very high up and I had the problem of passing a rubber stomach tube down the nostril to the stomach of a fidgety horse. Unfortunately the stepladders were a bit short and I had to stand on tip toes on the top step and several times fell off my perch, much to everyone's delight.

Life was new every day in the prairie. Off to castrate a colt in a paddock. I arrived to find that it was four-years-old and unhandled except for a lead rope and halter. I put the loop in the middle of a thirty foot rope around the restive horse neck. The two long ends were taken between the hind legs brought forward to the chest loop and then pulled tight bringing the hind legs up to the shoulder and the horse falls over. At this stage the horse can be tied up firmly and restrained. Unfortunately the horse had not read the instruction book and as the ropes touch his hind legs both feet struck out with a large crack and missed my head by inches. A direct hit and I would not have written this story.

We did not often get evening calls as it was beef country. About eight in the evening I was asked to see a cow about 20 miles north that had just calved and her uterus was falling out with the afterbirth. As all the roads were straight I arrived in good time and was directed to a patch of bush about half a mile distant.

I arrived to find the farmer equipped with a towel and water and prepared to sort out the problem. It was a beautiful warm evening and dusk was just descending. The prolapsed uterus was very rapidy sorted out but what I had not reckoned for was the constant bombardment by mosquitoes which seemed to scream down upon us like Stuka bombers. As we chatted at the end the farmer suddenly knocked me to the floor and waved us into silence. The newborn calf was wobbling around in the long grass nearby when a coyote looking for his evening meal appeared. Instantly the farmer reached into his shirt, pulled out a pistol and shot it.

At the start of October the first snow fell. It was forecast almost to the hour. We had four feet fall overnight. Fortunately I had plug heaters in the car and it started easily next morning. Another problem was that the tyres were a bit flat where they rested on the road and then froze in that state. Consequently the ride was a bit bumpetty until the rubber warmed up and they became round again.

After much industrious digging I cleared a passage to the road where the graders had been working throughout the night. This weather was where the practice's secret weapon came in useful. Bill had bought himself a three hundred horse power Bombardier. This was in reality a large wooden bodied vehicle to carry twelve people. It ran on tracks and had skids on the front that enabled it to go anywhere. He entered farms over the top of fences and even landed in one unit after driving over the top of the implement shed.

Unfortunately the medical services were also creating demands on its use. During the severe winter all tractors were put away in the shed and heavy horses used as transport. Many times I have ridden from the main road to the farm in the winter school bus. This consisted of small hut on skids pulled by the horse. Inside we were all snug in front of a wood fire.

Chapter Eighteen

THIS HAD BEEN ONE of the happiest times of my career as everything was constantly new. It was not very enjoyable for Margaret and Donal who were restricted without any transport, and they had little in common with the local people. As a result we decided to head for British Columbia and made some enquiries.

We contacted a vet, Trevor Clarkson, with a practice in Abbottsford in the Frazer Valley and went out to see him. We came to an agreement although I would be required to take a qualifying examination for the province. We arranged to join him later in the year.

Before leaving Neepawa I became involved in a slight comedy. Many of our calls on the prairie involved travelling up to one hundred miles but this was only forty miles distant. Jim Boyde had found a calf, at pasture, with a broken leg so could I call out to see him. I met him at the farm and he rode out into the bush where his Herefords were grazing. The calf in question was about two weeks old and carrying a broken foreleg. I managed to put on a splint and a light cast and he ran off to mammy complaining of his treatment.

Four weeks later I arranged for a revisit and returned to the site. The little calf was very well, thank you, and did not want us near him. As we approached he headed for the next county. And we pursued him across the pasture. I drove the VW Beetle with Jim standing on the seat whirling his lariat above the sunroof. We drove this way and that way trying in vain to loop the darned calf. He could corner like a speedway rider. Anyone watching would have thought that we were the Keystone cowboys. In the end Jim decided to leave it until another day.

Our first day in Abbotsford was an introduction to the farms in Sumas and Matsqui prairie in the Fraser Valley. It was a wide valley following the river and the road at that time had ribbon development along the 40 miles into Vancouver. This was changed shortly afterwards when the trans-Canada highway was developed.

The farming in the area was unlike anything that I had seen before. Most of the dairy herds were run by Dutch families. Farms were intensive due to the price of land, up to two hundred Holsteins, often on zero grazing.

The cows were housed in large sheds and lay in cubicles and never went out onto pasture. After milking they would be turned out in a yard or paddock to exercise and fed on sweetcorn silage and alfalfa hay. During wet spells their feet became sodden with water resulting in many foot problems. The milk yields from Holsteins were exceptionally high with many milk fever cases in new calvers. Trevor visited one farm and treated nine milk fevers in a row! Consequently the cows burnt themselves out early in life and never made old bones.

Due to the pressure put upon the cow herd by excessive milk production and mastitis there was always a lowered level of nutrition. Science was always running behind production levels. All cows were dosed with large magnets which lay in their stomachs for life and collected any metal which they ate, in particular, pieces of wire from the large alfalfa bales. This wire if left loose could penetrate the heart causing death.

Because of the stress put upon cows there was a fertility problem and the start of herd health visits to check up on pregnancy and low-grade disease problems.

Mastitis was a major problem as the cows often lay in unhygienic conditions. It was also a problem because there was unlimited access to antibiotic mastitis treatments. As a result the dairies had to resort to testing milk for antibiotics which interfered with cheese production and created antibiotic resistance in anyone drinking the milk, and in later years MRSA appeared as a consequence. All these situations were present in BC in 1960. It took them many years to arrive on Dartmoor.

I was having to look after Margaret and Donal increasingly as, much to our delight, she discovered that she was pregnant once again. Life was becoming a burden and I did more of the shopping. To complicate the situation I developed a rash on my arms and started to feel unwell. I ignored it for a few days and eventually decided to visit the doctor as I was having suicidal thoughts.

He examined me and said that he suspected that I had picked up brucellosis (Contagious Abortion) from a cow that I was calving. Several years before he had worked in the Peace River country, a long way from civilisation and received so many requests from local farmers that he bought a set of veterinary text books and instantly recognised the disease, which he confirmed by blood test.

I was fortunate in that he administered the correct treatment early on to prevent a long debilitating condition. Like many victims of brucellosis I became very depressed for about eight years. So now the roles were reversed as Margaret administered the TLC. It amazed me how she coped. Still as pretty as the day we married but carrying yet another bump.

One of our added pleasures was to see a rather eccentric character, complete with a flowing beard and flyaway hair, clad in striped shorts riding into town each day for his groceries. Apparently he would hitch his horse to a parking meter whilst he shopped and then ride back home again. It was rumoured that he also ran the local youth club! We met him personally after the house across the road was advertised for sale.

One evening there was a knock on the door and our bearded rider stood outside, dripping wet and in a state of shock. We took him in and lent him a dressing gown whilst Margaret took his sodden clothes off to be dried. Over a bottle of beer he told us his story. He was looking for new premises for his youth club and thought that he would look over the nearby house which was well lit by street lamps. He had opened an outhouse door where it was quite dark and as he stepped inside he fell into a well. Fortunately he was not hurt, only wet.

His other pursuit was creating a plan for world peace which he explained to us. He had sent copies to Winston Churchill, Einstein and the American president. Realising that he might be truly eccentric, I asked if I could see a copy of the document but unfortunately he did not have a spare available. Look what I missed out on!

I called into the surgery during the week and when I looked out of the window I was surprised to see a dead cougar hanging from a tree next door. Of course I had to examine it. It was very big and I found out that the next door neighbour was a game warden. It made me realise just how close we were to the wild country, particularly when I found that it had been shot within a mile of our house where the children played out in the garden

We were looking into the possibilities of settling in Canada permanently. After much thought regarding education and childhood we decided that we must return home. One of the main factors affecting us was that many Canadians had been reared in the poverty of the 1930s and felt that, with their current affluence, they must lavish everything upon their children from an early age.

Consequently, as they had not been reared in wartime England, it was automatic for children to be given expensive toys such as bikes just to 'keep up with the Jones's' and they had no period to hope for new presents and to save up for these items so they lost the excitement of anticipation. Starting off with little money creates a sense of values! This came home to us quite forcibly when it was reported that a young local couple fell out with their parents because they were not going to be given a furnished house for a wedding present!

The happy day arrived when Alison appeared. A beautiful little girl with cornflower blue eyes like her mother. Our world was complete with a pigeon pair. Donal was fascinated by the small snuffly creature who seemed to smile at all and sundry. As she started to sit up he would carry numerous toys to her just for her pleasure. As a result she didn't attempt to stand up until fifteen months of age.

When I called into the surgery one morning Trevor told me that my employment would cease from the following weekend 'because the Dutch farmers did not like me'. This came as a hammer blow as I had not received any complaints on my work and I thought I had an engaging personality.

As I received no other explanation I wondered whether this arose from my 'Englishness' as he had already exhibited that he had a chip on his shoulder regarding the UK. He had originated from humble origins which does leave some people embittered.

I had little money, so my first recourse was to speak to Gordon Thompson, the federal veterinarian who said that a brucellosis eradication programme was starting in the following week. He was no lover of Trevor, whom he regarded as being too keen on beer and finance, despite being an efficient veterinarian. "You watch and he will employ someone else shortly at a low salary until he is due to give him a rise." Sure enough four weeks later a new boy arrived in the practice. His presence didn't seem to affect my own work as I was hoping to practice on my own.

In the meantime I let it be known that I was setting up on my own with the help of the government blood testing income. After a short time work started to come in but I was having problems with disturbed nights and sleeplessness due to brucellosis. This increased my desire to return home although business was improving. Little did I realise that sleeplessness would be the pattern for the next eight years.

Chapter Nineteen

IN JUNE 1961 we returned to the UK and immediately carried out several locums in Formby. We stayed with Margaret's mum and it also gave me time to study the employment prospects in mixed practice.

There were quite a few vacancies, particularly in Wales, but I did not have language qualifications. So eventually we found a vacancy in a practice in Tavistock, on the edge of Dartmoor. This was an exciting prospect with cattle, sheep and horses in the area. This was to be a changing point in my career.

We left the children with Margaret's sister Gladys in Liverpool so that we could head off immediately for our overnight stay, 'The Rising Sun Hotel' in Lynmouth on the edge of Exmoor.

It was a beautiful crisp autumn day as we headed south through Cheshire towards our destination, through the Wye Valley and Bristol to follow our honeymoon route to Cornwall. It was a long drive in a small car and we eventually arrived at 'The Rising Sun' towards dusk.

After settling in our room we enjoyed a satisfying meal and sat in the lounge by an open fire. The walls were decorated with photographs of the horrifying flood which had swept through the village several years previously causing extensive damage and fatalities. Looking out of the window was a scene of tranquil beauty over the harbour with little evidence of residual damage.

We went for interview with Campbell Mackellar, a most unusual man. He was a very intelligent Scot who did not suffer fools gladly and could not stand still academically – 'Fame is the Spur'. He was a man driven by the urge to succeed in all he did! He knew exactly where he was going and how he was going to get there and was prepared to steam-roll those who stood in his path. He had joined the practice several years before, and succeeded the owner of the practice and pushed aside another colleague who did not measure up to his aims.

When we arrived, he and Anne, his wife made us very welcome into the six-man practice and explained what his aims were. His very incisive mind looked at all aspects of the practice and decided where improvements could take place. During the interview which took place at the Two Bridges hotel we were wined and dined by Campbell and Anne. He explained that this was the way to interview. Wives were always included as they were an essential part of the practice. On such occasions it was necessary to relax to assess the situation. In vino, veritas!

The practice worked from two small rooms and a garage in a side street. The operating room, about eight feet by eight feet had white-washed walls and ceiling with cobwebbed windows. The skill required during small animal surgery was to lean across the patient to avoid flakes of whitewash from the ceiling falling into the wound. New premises were in plans for the future!

One of the greatest assets of the practice was Bill Cackett who had started many years before as the coachman and general dogsbody. He could talk to anyone, had an in depth knowledge of the practice clients and organised drug dispensing and compounding, which made him a valued member of the business.

The sheep department needed improving. Individual visits to farms for lambings were uneconomical for farmer and vet — much better to have lambing facilities at the surgery. When I arrived one vet was in the surgery all day from 15th February for six weeks delivering lambs or carrying out caesareans. The first caesarean took twenty five minutes and the third one up to an hour as fatigue set in.

Therefore a cup of coffee between operations speeded up service. Old broken-mouthed ewes with irregular teeth had their teeth ground down, which gave them an extra productive year. Vasectomies in rams were treated likewise-at the surgery

Those vets who were on night call might have to visit the surgery two or three times during the night to attend to lambings. A number of the farmers would return from the pub at closing time and then go out to check on the sheep at pasture. They would then be able to call on the 'vetinry' in the early hours of the morning just after he had staggered off to bed.

A similar self-discipline affected the cattle side of the practice, whether it was dairy or beef breeds. We had several large dairy herds and the beef mainly consisted of South Devon cattle, the 'gentle giants' of the cattle world. They are a wonderful breed to handle unless they lean or fall on you. The milk is yellowish and high in butterfat and the beef is marbled.

In other words the fat is interspersed through the muscle and not in lumps in the meat.

The greatest problem encountered in cattle was babesiais or redwater transmitted by ticks on acidic pastures. The disease is passed on by a tick bite and the parasite develops in the blood cells causing them to rupture and blood appears in the urine.

The onset of the disease can be extremely rapid. Having been seen in the morning the animal can be dead by evening if left untreated. An injection can effect a cure although acute anaemia can result and requires treatment using blood transfusion from a healthy or immune animal.

The most efficient means of control was for the farmer to check his cattle twice daily and dress the pastures with lime to reduce acid levels. Raking over the pasture also broke down the moist microclimate which suited the ticks.

It was not uncommon for us to transfuse three animals in a day to combat the disease.

The surgery had a large number of citrated bottles ready to take onto the farm at any time for transfusions. Science moved on and these bottles were superseded by human urine bags which were much more convenient to carry and use.

One of the great problems of living in South Devon cattle country was obstetrics. There are several breeds of cattle, Charollais and Belgian Blue which have these common drawbacks but they also have the asset of producing the most appetising beef. The problem is over-development of muscle (double-muscling) in the calves which prevents normal birth and requires caesarian section.

All these difficulties intrigued Campbell's enquiring mind and he investigated them in detail and he wrote many papers on the subject. His enthusiasm spilled out onto the rest of the practice so that each member who attended a calving was required to take measurements of the calf and record their weight. All this data was included in

Campbell's academic papers. This was a labour of love to us as we were contributing to new research.

A further contribution that South Devon cattle made to our work was that a percentage of them prolapsed their uterus after calving. This is a delightful condition where the uterus is forced out of the body and we would be called out to put it back into place. Often this happens early in the morning. The cow may be lying out at pasture, recumbent with milk fever and in the pouring rain or snow.

The uterus would be liberally covered with mud and cow dung. After washing the organ well with soap and warm water it was suspended on a clean sheet of plastic sheet so that one could push this enormous mass, weighing about 80 pounds, back inside.

As it was always swollen and congested with blood, several drugs had to be given to try and reduce its size and it was liberally sprinkled with six pounds of sugar to absorb the fluids. This procedure was very tiring even for the fittest young vets.

It was my turn next. Each year we met quite a number of cases of bracken poisoning. This is a fatal and distressing condition in cattle and Campbell suggested that I should look into the effects of our current treatments on the disease. I took this up with great enthusiasm but was eventually delighted when an academic in Wales produced a paper disproving all the work I had done as I was floundering in my investigation.

Campbell's enthusiasm knew no bounds. Each evening when we finished surgery at 6p.m. he would arrive in the office and, seeing that we were quite tired, would say "Would you like to share a wee dram across in the Market Inn, laddie?"

This was one of his ploys to have some mental exercise with his employees. It was his version of mental press-ups! His initial comments would always be to ask my opinion on certain conditions. If I stumbled in my response he would say that I should do more reading to keep up.

After a month or two it suddenly dawned on me that when I was consulting, he would be reading up the latest information in the Veterinary Journals and using them as ammunition to quiz me. Eventually I would read up academic articles in textbooks and put them to him along the counter of the Market Inn.

He would go quite silent whilst he lit another Woodbine and reply "Well that's as may be laddie" and add that it was my turn to buy a round. We both enjoyed this mental jousting which kept us mentally on our toes.

One evening he asked me if I would like to go to a veterinary meeting the next day in Beaulieu, but we must set off early in the morning. I replied that I should be delighted but what was it about?

"Well, it's a talk on blood transfusion in cattle which might help when I write my observations and there are several people I want to speak to on veterinary politics."

Of course I was delighted to keep him company as it was nearly a four-hour drive. What I did not realise was that I was being used! He was really probing to find out how useful I might be in the future.

He later confided in me that friends were there to be used, which did not fit in with my outlook in life. His life was completely dominated by academic pursuit and veterinary politics.

At home Anne ran the household, reared the children (as he could become irascible in the presence of screaming, shouting, fighting little boys) and she kept a well-equipped toolbox for repairs throughout the house. She had to be a mother and father figure.

As we drove into Hampshire he told me that his life expectancy was about 56 years as both his parents had died at that age and he expected to die then too. Suddenly all was revealed. This drive to succeed was based on this premise; the Woodbines and whisky were fuel to the fire of his ambition. It was a case of 'Fame is the Spur'. He had to feel important to attain his goal in life. After Anne's death his sons asked me to tell them about Campbell as they knew nothing about him as a person.

During the next year a site was found for the new premises, opposite the Cattle Market Inn, ensuring a constant flow of farmers during the market days. I took great interest in its development and of course the pub was an ideal site for us to exchange ideas on construction.

In hindsight the small animal department appeared to be very inadequate. We had an operating theatre, two kennels and four cat cages. To us, at that time, this was ideal and we looked forward to a growing clientele as most of the local small animal work went to Plymouth.

Here again Campbell demonstrated his ability to think laterally. At that time the Royal College of Veterinary Surgeons would not permit advertising. A veterinary practice could have a brass plate at the door, no greater than nine inches by twelve inches with the name of the practice.

Campbell had already built up a network of influential friends in the profession and could rely on their backing. He arranged a formal opening of the premises by Lord Roborough, who happened to be Lord Lieutenant of Devon, and also had the BBC from Plymouth to show the ceremony on television. All the arrangements were carried out quietly and the Western Morning News was also present. Any complaints from the veterinary governing body were very muted as the Queen's representative had taken part in the opening ceremony. Fait accompli!

The Ministry of Agriculture in Exeter had recently been insisting that if the practice carried out TB tests on farms and any other work on the farm (or any nearby farms), then the entire mileage should be charged to the farmer and not to the government. This did not go down well with the farmer or ourselves.

The government offices would not discuss the situation so the problem rumbled on for a long time until the MAFF, in a fit of pique, stopped sending testing to our practice, as a result of which the farmers never 'found it convenient to have cattle available' on the appointed day. Eventually common sense prevailed and the bullying ceased. This made an indelible impression on my attitude to government departments where the cult of persecution still prevails.

In June 1963 we were blessed with our third child, another blue-eyed little girl, Kathleen. Our cup was full to brimming! She was no trouble to anyone and she had a brother and sister on call to supply her wants.

Oft times our practice relations could become strained, perhaps as a result of my light-hearted approach to life – I was born with my cup half full! Only Campbell was permitted to carry out treatment on the mink farm. I never worked out why but I suspect that it gave him a feeling of importance.

One day he rushed through the surgery to his office. I was talking to a client across the counter. As he sped through there came a curt query "What's the dosage of Gonadotrophin for mink?" Without turning I responded. "Fifteen hundred international units, Campbell" as if I used it daily.

Twenty minutes later, when I had imagined that he had been looking up the information, he suddenly reappeared looking slightly puzzled.

"How in the hell did you know that."

"Easy!" I responded. "You had no idea, so my guess was more accurate." Suddenly his lips went straight as he had one of those disapproving fits and he slammed into his office.

Like many strongly opinionated people he could have a 'down' on someone who was a bit reticent. He walked in one day and said to me

"I have the annual bonuses arranged. Except for Tony."

"Why," I replied, "I think he's worked jolly hard and deserves one." Irritated by my defiance of his decision he continued, "Well in that case you won't need one either."

Despite our tiffs we worked very well together. On New Year's Eve 1963, the cold winter descended on Dartmoor. We awoke to a silent snowbound landscape, nothing moved. The snow lay thick on the ground, the sky was leaden and the trees decorated with cotton wool. Fortunately I was equipped with snow chains and managed to reach the surgery.

Campbell had already had a call to a milk fever at Roborough and we both set off in the Land Rover plus a toboggan and milk crate loaded with empty bottles. As the milkman would not appear for a couple of days and we were heading to a dairy farm, we hoped to supply the firm with milk. We followed a snowplough leading an ambulance to the maternity ward in Plymouth.

There were no other calls that day as everyone was busy combating the weather. We had to walk a mile though snowdrifts to treat the patient. Having done that we loaded up twelve lemonade bottles with milk and towed them on the toboggan back to the car. We arrived back in town to silence as few cars had ventured forth.

I hurried back to the house to a scene of chaos. The milk was welcome but we had no water and no lunch. All the water pipes to our first storey flat had been laid two inches below the surface and had frozen solid. Fortunately our neighbours below had water and, understanding our predicament that children require lots of water, offered to send it up by hosepipe. By this means we had a bath full of water and coils of green hosepipe, and the kids bathed in the kitchen sink for the next six weeks. The children loved their first snow and had great fun tobogganing down the garden.

As a result of the big freeze our work

dropped dramatically. In many cases it was impossible for the farmers to reach their stock although they did struggle out with hay. Hundreds of sheep and lambs were lost in snowdrifts. Where do you start to search on the vastness of the moor? Possibly, on the 'hirsels' where the sheep preferred to graze. Many problems were eased when the army flew hay out in helicopters and had fodder drops near groups of cattle or ponies. Being the smallest in the practice Ken Sanders was sent off on one flight to near Princetown in order to deliver triplets to a cow.

Princetown was cut off by road for six weeks which made it completely upset the plans of any prisoners planning a New Year break out. The majority of them were too busy caring for the needs of the cattle and pigs on the farm whilst others kept local roads and footpaths clear.

Back at the surgery life moved very slowly as the small animal clients were few and far between. A lot of time was taken up developing our skills at playing poker. A very good cure for boredom!

As the conditions improved we were increasingly involved in farm visits, treating many animals debilitated through the severe weather. Magnesium and molasses licks were used to prevent the onset of 'Grass Staggers' as the growth of grass had been set back by the cold. The shutdown of necessary nutrition for in-lamb ewes triggered off 'twin lamb disease' so we were greeted by many stupid sheep staring blindly into space. Mortality was high in affected animals and nutritional support helped the rest of the flock.

The springtime resulted in lower lambing averages followed by a rainy few months and increase in Redwater due to the humid conditions. That year, possibly due to stress of the winter on the cattle and the wet spring, we had an increase in the number of redwater cases occurring.

Campbell was the great lateral thinker and, shortly after I joined him, we had a committee meeting in the Market Inn when he announced that he was concerned that many of the moor farmers were slow payers and so he had worked on a plan to improve our cash flow. "There's no way I can pay good salaries to you laddies unless the farmers settle their bills. From the end of this month we shall give a discount of five per cent on all accounts paid within 30 days, but before that I shall increase our charges by seven and a half per cent. Not only that laddie, we must arrange a reasonable scale of fees across the day and stop these farmers from sitting in the pub all evening and then calling us out towards midnight. The cheapest calls will be those sent in during the morning. An increased charge in the afternoon and a bit more in the evening. An extra charge should occur after eleven p.m." With a smirk of satisfaction he bought us all a drink before going home.

Later in the week he told us that he had talked to the Spooner's Hunt committee about their annual show. "Previously we have attended the show as a part of our duty but I feel that the time has come to be realistic and charge a fee. When I explained that I had to pay you to attend or give cover they reluctantly agreed, particularly as we vaccinate the hounds at cost price."

He was involved in a group, S.P.V.S., who felt that the profession should evaluate its charges uniformly throughout the country instead of the internecine squabbling and undercutting that took place between many veterinary practices. For better or for worse he helped to pull the profession into the modern era.

At this stage Campbell was climbing the ladder of success. He would announce to us that he was off to give a talk to one of the veterinary societies across the country on one of his favourite subjects on which he had written a paper. These included Redwater in cattle, blood transfusion in cattle or the causes of oversize calves in South Devon cows. As he was skilled at networking, it was not long he was picked as Devon representative on the Council of the British Veterinary Association.

Such was his thirst for knowledge that we were always being encouraged, nay driven, to look into various aspects of animal disease worth researching. After my failure to find a cure for Bracken poisoning he suggested that I look into the factors causing yellow fat in some breeds of sheep but unfortunately I had to leave the practice when this project was about to start. (However I did eventually follow my dream and study for a Master's degree in fish diseases.) Bit of a non-sequitur

During my stay in Devon I joined two other practice for short periods in my search for a perfect partnership. One in Kingsteignton and one in Poole, Dorset. I left the Poole

practice because it was rapidly becoming solely small animal and there was quite a lot of friction amongst the neighbouring small animal practices.

The Kingsteignton practice had three centres and very little co-ordination between the vets concerned. I returned to Tavistock at the request of Campbell, on the basis that I could be offered a partnership in the near future as David Juby was emigrating to New Zealand. I was delighted to return to an organised practice but had doubts about taking up the partnership. Campbell was too focused on his aims, and at some stage I could see a parting of the ways.

He needed reliable people around him as he had become vice-president of the British Veterinary Association, which would involve a lot of time at meetings in London. His main problem was that he had picked up a persistent virus – we later found this to be brucellosis, so I realised that he could be in for a period of depression for several years similar to my own problem!

Whilst I was there we also went off to support the newly-formed Cornwall Veterinary Association where I became involved in the committee organising their stand at the Royal Cornwall Show in June.

In due course Margaret and I were called to the show stand erection day when all committee members and children worked hard all day and finished up with a picnic, as we put the finishing touches to our exhibit. This involved a lot of fellowship and I found my colleagues in Cornwall to be very welcoming.

I also met David Gethin, who told me that he was leaving the practice in Helston and heading for Africa. When I enquired, he said that there would be a vacancy for an assistant in September and he gave me the details of the owner Charlie Head. David gave me information on the practice and from my viewpoint it appeared to be eminently suitable. When I explained the situation to Margaret she was enthusiastic as she felt it was about time that we finally settled down after working in seven practices.

Chapter Twenty

SOON AFTER THE SHOW in June we arranged to meet Charles and Elvera Head and drove down to Helston to see them on a Sunday morning. They lived in a splendid stone built house, covered with Virginia creeper in the centre of Helston. It was called Coinage Hall as it had once been the assay house for the local tin mines. We were fortunate at a later date to find the old assay papers from the mines lying in the roof space.

The door was opened by Elvera Head, a silver-haired lady with a welcoming smile. "You will be Margaret and Noel, come in and meet my Charlie – he's mowing the lawn!"

She led us into the kitchen and called Charles in from the garden. He was tall, about six feet five inches and ruddy faced. He walked with a limp, which we were led to understand was memento of the war in Sicily. He had a commanding presence and was very much an army officer.

He greeted us warmly. "We're glad to see you both. The practice could do with some young blood since my partner died several years ago. David spoke well of you. Of course we shall miss his enthusiasm.

"I know that V has a lovely lunch prepared for you when we can sit down and discuss business. What'll you drink old boy, and of course Margaret."

We lunched in the large sunlit kitchen and seemed to chat away for a long time about farming and large animal practice. This was a practice which had been run by his father and grandfather so the family had been involved in the area for some sixty years. Charles had fought with the commandos during the war and had many amazing stories to tell.

"Don't expect me to get involved in small animal practice," continued Charles. "I know nothing about it and can't stand many of the owners."

"Don't worry" I responded. "I have lots of energy and if you would like me to build up the pet side I am happy to take any calls"

"Thanks old boy. At present we have one other assistant who is quite young and our son John is at London Vet College at present – due to qualify in 1972, if he gets through his exams! In the meanwhile I will offer John Saunders and yourself a partnership in two years 'as long as we see eye-to-eye'. I want to take it a bit easier as I am getting older and goodness knows V deserves a bit of rest. "The large animal side of the practice consists of family-owned farms that you will get on with if you enjoyed Dartmoor. The large animal side can increase and as the small animal work is zero David tells me that there is much that we can do."

We chatted away happily as Charles drove us around the area and we were delighted with Porthleven and the nearness of the sea. V kept pointing out points of interest and was such a charming host that she could well have been a

West Cornwall publicity officer. After a lovely cream tea we set off home after promising to phone Charlie during the next few days with a decision on his offer.

As we headed towards Dartmoor we discussed the day's outing and found a common bonding towards the offer. "I think that Charles is a man whose word is his bond, I said. " He is not high powered but just wishes to continue his way of life and care for his clients who are an extended family. He will encourage us to develop the practice without worrying about research and setting goals as Campbell does!"

"I agree" continued Margaret. "He is a man's man and definitely happy in his life style and he has the great asset of being married to Elvera who runs his life and could charm the birds from the trees. I really took to her bubbly personality."

After settling down in Tavistock once more we weighed up the pros and cons during the next few days. We settled for Helston and I handed in my three months notice to Campbell. I did feel guilty as he still had problems with brucellosis and I had very much to thank him for in teaching me how to run a practice and the intellectual benefits of research. We were also going to miss the company of Ken and Jenny Sanders, Harry and Mary Cummings and the many farming friends we had met. Every private wants to be a sergeant and I was aiming for an equitable partnership.

I had already become involved with a fish veterinary group organised by Mary Brancker, a past president of BVA and John Mace, one of the first British vets involved in fish medicine. This group was developed to cope with the increasing number of fish farms which had sprung up over the country and I felt that I would like to contribute as one of my early dreams had been to study fish medicine. This dream was getting nearer as a fish disease course had started in Stirling and, if the time and finances were right, I would love to study there.

We arrived in Helston in October 1968 with the aid of Harry and Mary to move our furniture. Elvera had organised a house for us to stay overwinter at Parc-an-Fold farm in Mawgan.

Our first two weeks were very noisy as the house lay under the helicopter flight path for Culdrose Naval station but the sound gradually faded into the background as we acclimatised to it. Very soon we learnt that Cornwall is at the bottom of the scale salary-wise but excels in goodwill. I had never seen so many Bond minicar three-wheelers. This mattered little as many Cornish folk rarely ventured beyond Plymouth. Everywhere we went we were welcomed.

The next step was to organise my car with drugs and equipment as each practice differs in its approach It had already been decided that as soon as I was free from farm calls that I should make myself available to organise the non-existent small animal side of the practice.

As soon as I arrived I met Carna Basset, the receptionist, who organised the calls and handed out drugs. She passed me on to Stuart Williams who was animal nurse, general factotum and the handyman around the premises. We hit it off at once because we had many common interests on the animal side.

Stuart was able to locate most of the equipment for my car, which had previously been used by David Gethin. I had also many ideas of my own and we set off around the town buying waders and ropes. On our return he introduced me to Bert Hichens who had been with the practice most of his life. Like Bill Cackett in Tavistock, he could mix up many of the medicines and of course knew many of the local clients by name and history.

He was a little old man dressed up in a battered old suit and a cap which was a permanently on his head. He had already retired twice but kept coming back to work as he knew nothing else. Possibly one incentive was that he was given an old coat each time he resigned.

One of his most valued assets was his old battered cap which kept the sun out of his eyes and enabled him to scan the ground in front as he shuffled up the street. He never missed a coin that had fallen in the road or gutter and he would swoop upon it and slip it into his pocket. I suspected that he had a large stash of money hidden away under his bed.

At this stage I met John Saunders, the other assistant, who rushed in and out again in a hurry to get out on the farm to get the day's work done and get back again. He was very slimly built, dark haired with a moustache and heavy glasses and lived in the small practice house 'Chy Vean' with his wife Hilde and two sons. I later found that his whole life was lived at a frenetic rate due to his excitable temperament. He had no ability to deal with small animals or their owners due to his nature. Even in his car he drove with his foot flat on the accelerator.

His greatest fault was not understanding the Cornish expression 'dreckly' which typifies the Cornish outlook and indicates something slower than the Spanish 'manăna'!

John could not wait for matters to resolve themselves and had to keep pushing. (We had one local smallholder who milked ten cows, starting 10am and then again at 10 pm. This did cause a problem when he requested a visit at 10.30p.m.) It upset his stamp collecting.

John's all absorbing interest was philately. He was quite an authority on German stamps and had acquired a fairly valuable collection which made my simple collecting appear to be very amateur. Any of my spare time was involved in trout fishing or attending veterinary functions to meet my colleagues in the county.

Once I had my car organised I set off, with Stuart to guide me for a couple of days. My first visit was to a South Devon cow at Trenoon which was overdue to calve. Alarm bells started to ring. "Have we got a caesarian kit handy Stuart?" I queried. "Not exactly," responded Stuart, "David carried out our only caesarean operation about six months ago! But we seem to have lots of forceps and needles in the drawer."

"Let's collect them all together," I said. "Perhaps Mrs Head has an old sauce pan to boil up the tools and I shall look around for suture materials, anyway I have lots of fishing line. Perhaps you could come to guide and assist me as I don't know my way around Mullion."

Together we headed off to the farm and found the heifer in a loose box with the head and toes of the calf just showing. The calf's head was swollen and it was evidently dead. The heifer was as fat as a butterball and no doubt this was part of the problem – too much internal fat and an overgrown calf.

As the calf was partly out we decided that surgery would only cause more problems and a lot of expense so with Mr Gilbert's consent Stuart and I set to work use traction with a calving aid and lots of lubrication to ease the journey of the foetus. The heifer was quite torn and exhausted by the end of our work and the calf had been dead over twenty four hours.

As we had a cup of tea afterwards I suggested to George that he kept his heifers on short rations for the last six weeks of pregnancy so that they would not be so fat and the calves would be smaller. He thought for a moment and, with a welcoming smile, replied, "I suppose that I should really but they always look so pretty and contented when they are nice and round." I guessed that I was never going to win this battle. Strangely enough he must have considered the situation as his calving problems seemed to ease off.

There were quite a few South Devon herds in the area and the farmers were delighted to have a vet who loved and understood the breed. There did not appear to be so many calving problems as in Tavistock, which I put down to different bulls in the area and one very knowledgeable breeder Wallis Williams.

He was a small curly-haired man in his fifties with a whimsical sense of humour who was always pipe smoking, and was liable to disappear in a thick cloud of tobacco smoke as he considered my questions.

He had three sons, one a specialist pig breeder, one who carried out arable work and the third who helped with the South Devon herd. Wallis was much in demand as a South Devon judge and had travelled as far as South Africa.

It took me some time to understand the farming colloquialisms such as 'she refused her meat or her flour' really meant that she wasn't eating. A troublesome cow was not a problem but she was in season and ready to "steal the bull!"

Shortly after I arrived I was invited to join a Young Farmers Quiz panel and I was selected to answer the first question. 'Could I advise the audience on the best way to make sweet hay'. I made an earnest attempt to go through the preparation of hay and then to my embarrassment found out that it was a local expression for rolling in the hay fields with your sweetheart.

The Lizard Peninsula and surrounding area were devoted to family-run dairy farms and small holdings with cropping and pig enterprises. It was a time of self-sufficiency and the country folk were happy with their lot in a beautiful county where life was still comparatively slow.

Soon after I arrived, however, I was introduced to 'Daisy'. I was greeted by Stuart one morning with the comment that we must go and visit 'Daisy'. "Great!" I replied, "Is she a dog or one of a milking herd?"

He answered me with a slow Cornish smile. "Not 'xactly, Daisy is an eight-foot alligator who lives in the kitchen, and we regularly have to force feed her when the weather is cold."

Now the Cornish have a delightful sense of humour. I had learned to be wary in replying. "Tell me a bit more Stuart. Is this a big leg-pull?" He looked deeply hurt and said "No! David and I used to go out to see old Mrs Roberts regularly to sort out the problem. Ask Carna! He said defensively. "Daisy won't eat you. You're a bit old and tough."

"Let's go! What gear do I need ? Ropes and bull holders"

"Not really. You might consider that the power of prayer is useful in some cases," he responded with a quiet smile. "Let's head for Tregarne Mill where the full fairy story will unfold."

We headed off to St Keverne and followed the road to Tregarne Mill which lay down in a deep valley, surrounded by trees. Stuart jumped out of the car and pulled on his thigh boots. Did we have to enter a swamp to greet the patient?

As we entered the front door I was greeted by Mrs Roberts who emerged from the slate flagged kitchen. She was old and bent, wearing a time-worn floral pinafore, and moving with the aid of a stick. "Hello Mr Stuart, we're glad you could come as Daisy has not eaten for days and I should hate her to starve. I'm glad that Stuart Williams has come as he knows Daisy well."

She led us into the kitchen where I saw Daisy, in a six-foot galvanised tank. She was feeling rather disgruntled at having her mobility ramp removed and water emptied away. Daisy, eight feet of alligator, dark green and black with shiny teeth protruding each side of her jaws and slit eyes looking through me, was summing me up as a culinary delicacy. I, of course, was quietly conversing with my Maker putting my future into His hands asking for strength and the agility of a deer.

Help was at hand as Ma Roberts handed me a broomstick with a cloth padded end, saying, "Don't worry Mr Stuart! I always feed her either calf's heart or boned chicken to stop any bones puncturing her tummy. Stuart kneels astride Daisy and holds her head steady. I hold her jaws open and you throw in her food to the back of the throat and push it down her gullet."

With the air of a conjuror, I was handed a piece of chicken whilst she bent down to Daisy muttering and prising her jaws open, "Come along my darling. Take your nice dickie bird!" I threw the chicken in and pushed it gently down her throat before standing back to admire my handy work. "Thanks God! We did a good job there." Stuart stood up and we went off to wash our hands in a rather basic and grubby sink.

Mrs Roberts gratefully said, "Thank you! We'll see you in three days as she always goes off food in cool weather." Then it occurred to me that of course, being a reptile she is poikilothermic and would slip into a state of torpor in cold conditions. I called back in three days and could see a busy time ahead.

I had to visit Daisy regularly over a period of months, which opened my eyes to her checkered past. Daisy had appeared in five films including "In the Dog House" and "An alligator called Daisy". For the first five years she was called "Peter" – until she laid an egg.

The first few months in Helston were fascinating in that it was a damp, misty autumn, so that by Christmas time I had not been able to appreciate the beauties of the coastline as everywhere was continually clad in fog. The story was that this incessant misty weather had persuaded the navy to change from fixed wing to flying helicopters from Culdrose. By the time of our arrival it was the main helicopter training base for NATO. One airfield on The Lizard had been used by Barnes Wallis in his experiments on the 'bouncing bomb' for the Dam Busters raid.

We were so fortunate to find a house for sale in a third of an acre between the town and the schools. This was an ideal situation with a garden to satisfy Margaret's 'green fingers' passion, a large, tiered rock garden and fruit trees and two lawns for the children. This was heaven so far as we were concerned. The garden was almost surrounded with stone walls which could contain dogs, cats and children. We had entered another stage of our journey.

It is easy to be complacent and say that this was another step in my vocation but there were still challenges to meet. Like Don Quixote I must seek further challenges in life and windmills with which to joust.

Once we had settled in our nest I felt a compulsion to meet my colleagues in this friendly county. I attended many local veterinary meetings and, of course, the veterinary stand at the annual county show. Confrontation amongst colleagues in the county was almost unknown and within three years I felt that we could address everyone by their Christian names over a cup of coffee.

Many of the farms were very small and I used to treat several small holdings where the stock amounted to four cattle. These were cherished pets and should not be handled roughly. Each had a name and birth date. The cows were hand milked to supply the owners and neighbours whilst the excess fed the suckling calf and maybe an adopted calf if she was milking well.

I was called in to one holding where the average age of the stock was ten years. The two cows were so fat that they could not become pregnant. The other two stock were steers who were absolute butter balls. Just pets!

To demonstrate the speed of life I received a call to a calving on one gentle summer's evening. Jack Lethbridge had run beef South Devon all his life and as the years rolled by his herd reduced in size to meet his energy quotient. I arrived at his small-holding about seven in the evening. It had been a warm day and the sky was bright blue as the sun was lowering over the verdant pasture.

"I'm a bit worried about old Bessie, Mr Stuart, as she's kept thin despite the good grazing. She's been standing in the corner for several hours making a few attempts to calve and then gives up, like she's tired. I'll just drive her in to the loose-box where I can tie her up!"

I got all my gear together whilst he went off to collect the statutory pail of warm water, soap and a towel. I inserted my arm into her uterus. All I could feel was afterbirth and a small calf ready to be born. "Hold on Jack this appears to be quite easy! I can't imagine why she's not got on with it." With a gentle pull a pretty little heifer was soon on the straw, kicking and spluttering. I checked her and there, down low, was a second small calf ready to join her sibling.

"I'll just check her for milk fever or mastitis to see what's causing the problem as she's looking bright enough. I don't really know why she's so lazy!"

"Could it be her age!" commented Jack.

"Tell me?" I responded.

"I was working out the other evening that she's about twenty two years old," he said "This is her third set of twins!"

"This is her last calving!" I responded. "You're not being fair to her and carrying a calf is too much. How old was your wife when she had her last child?"

"About thirty-five, I suppose. Now I see what you're getting at. Actually, I didn't mean for her to get in calf but she 'stole the bull' when I wasn't lookin'. Mind you he was so young that I didn' think he was up to it."

"Right I'll leave you to look after her and call in in a few days to check that she's not out stealing bulls again!" I continued chuckling at the thought of old Bessie having a gigolo!

Pets also add to the joys of practice as many of them are child replacements or a sop to the owner's feelings of inadequacy. Some of my most intensive dealings have taken place with young married couples whose pet is the centre of their life until a child arrives and the pet rightly drops down the pecking order.

Often a dominant partner can also interfere with case histories or treatment. I recall well the first consultation from a new client who initially enquired whether I was capable of treating pedigree Siamese cats who had won many rosettes at shows. Fortunately, my excellent receptionist confirmed that I was the Siamese expert in the practice and would have all the answers to her troubles.

When the time came, Mrs Thomasina Timberlake and her husband arrived with the patients. Mrs T was a big handsome lady who delighted in power dressing. She swept into the surgery like a sailing ship in full sail. "Oh Mr Stuart", she gushed. "I spoke to Dr Andrews, President of the Cat Fancy. She recommended you very highly as you talk to the cats and are so gentle."

She turned to her husband who had struggled in with two large baskets. It was rather like Jack Sprat as he was small and skinny and peered out from beneath a large flat cap. Pushing him aside Thomasina commanded: "George! Do hurry up with the boys, Mr Stuart is a busy man and can't wait all day. She opened the cages and extracted two rather skinny Siamese cats who appeared rather alarmed at their treatment.

"Oh! Mr Stuart these are my two boys, Peter and Paul, who take up so much of our lives, don't they George!" said Thomasina. "They are not very well, but I can't put my finger on the problem. They are such sensitive creatures and could have picked up a virus during the stormy weather. Do you think that it could be caused by living near the coast?"

"I heard them coughing and one had diarrhoea early this morning," interjected George. Inflating herself she retorted loudly. "Don't be silly George. There has not been a sniffle between them."

"No dear!" said George in a tone often adopted by the long-suffering. The two cats stood on the examination table unsure as to whether they should be ill or not. Listening to Peter's lungs I could hear very faint sounds and decided to treat him. Whilst I injected him he stoically accepted his treatment. Then I realised that he was not very gifted mentally – the scrambled brain syndrome seen in some strains of Siamese.

Paul, however, was a clumsy Siamese. He walked around the consulting room stumbling over every small object such as stethoscope, small boxes and shoes etcetera. I was quite concerned for his vision if let outside.

"Mrs Timberlake I am quite concerned about Paul's vision. It does require checking and we are fortunate to have a consultant in Tavistock who could satisfy your concerns. I can contact him and arrange for you to take the boys along together for examination as there might be a familial problem.

"An excellent idea Mr Stuart. Do speak to him as soon as possible. George," she commanded in her normal haughty manner, "put the boys back in their baskets and take them to the car." True to his duty, George scuttled off with the unfortunate cats.

Within three weeks we received a report to the effect that Paul was partially blind and Peter also affected. They were the result of poor breeding.

The next time that I met Mrs Timberlake she was a changed person. George had died suddenly and she had lost nearly five stone in weight as she crept into the surgery, a little old lady. She had lost her crutch to lean on and had nobody to dominate.

How many times do we hear about dog attacks – some fatal? These are often the property of owners who are quite small in stature or intellect. They love to strut about with a potentially aggressive dog to give themselves a feeling of power. Gang members in the cities build themselves up with steroids and thrive on rearing such animals to develop their aggression where they can also be used as bodyguards or in a dog-fighting arena. This condition is known as LMS, the 'little man syndrome' and is evident in dictators such as Stalin, Mussolini, Hitler and Putin.

Discipline is an essential in all animals as they can revert to 'the pack' state, unless supervised. How many times each year is it reported that family pets have attacked and killed children due to lack of direct supervision?

One of my early meetings with Cornish farmers involved Joe and Elaine Lane who farmed at Higher Lanner. They were having problems with their rabbit farming enterprise which was the latest get-rich-quick fad to hit the farming world.

I set off to Higher Lanner with little knowledge of rabbit medicine and less of Cornish farmers. As I drove into the yard Joe walked out of the house to greet me. He was a well-built cheerful man wearing a flat cap. "You'll be Noel Stuart. I've heard some good reports on you and I hear that you enjoy a pint of Spingo at the Blue Anchor! Better come and have a look in this shed where Elaine keeps her rabbits. She reckons that we've been losin' money too long and they rabbits could make us a fortune.

We entered the low hut to see rows of rabbit pens each with a plump rabbit and a litter. You could have cut the urine-filled air with a knife as all the windows were tight shut.

"Let's have some air in here Joe, lest they all die of pneumonia. I'll bet that you have more air circulating in your piggery. Several seem to have mastitis and diarrhoea. There is quite a problem with your husbandry."

"I'm glad you said that", retorted Joe in his slow country manner. "I think that Elaine's ideas of livestock keeping have slipped a bit. I wouldn't like that atmosphere in my piggery, too much ammonia from stale urine. Come on in and see the lady. She has a pot of tea handy."

As we entered the airy kitchen Elaine welcomed us with a table spread with cake and a pot of tea. She was a small, smiley person with a fresh complexion.

"Sit down and tell me the worst Mr Stuart. Why are we getting these problems with the rabbits. It all seemed so simple when the man called to talk to us about it although we hear that they have had lots of problems at the 'Nonsuch' Farm unit."

"It's like this," I replied. "Did the salesman go through the finances with you and put forward a business plan? The old shed has not got good enough ventilation because the ventilation holes are stuffed with straw and you have a build-up of urine in there. He supplied you with feed pellets which I suspect contain too much protein and too little fibre. This gives them lots of profit, and I suspect that if your cows were on a comparable feed they would suffer in the same way."

Joe and Elaine sat listening wide eyed. "Well the way you put it maybe he didn't go into it thoroughly. You see we're simple and not too educated. The way we tell if we are making money is to go into the bank and see if the account is increasing or droppin' "

"Well, I would get on to them and advise the company to take back the rabbits if they don't improve. Otherwise you will keep losing money and have big veterinary bills. I'll call back in a couple of days to follow the story"

I drove off feeling quite satisfied and told my story to Carna back in the office. She chuckled and said that Elaine had been a smart cashier in the bank and was no fool with money and I had fallen for the Lane's leg-pulling technique. "They dearly love to have a bit of fun at your expense and you walked right into it." replied Carna. "You'll know for next time. They both love a joke if they think that you are too serious."

I did enjoy Joe's company, as I never knew what to expect from this large, shambling man from one day till the next. I was calling to see one of his Ayrshire cows one beautiful sunny morning when he appeared out of the piggery door. He waved me in. "Come and see Belinda (named after his mother-in-law) this Lop Eared sow of mine. She has just had her first litter by artificial insemination."

I stood and admired the litter of thirteen piglets happily suckling their mother who was grunting contentedly. "How do you do it Joe? Does the artificial inseminator call round when she is in season?"

"Naithin' like that. I went off on an insemination course and brought back the straws full of semen which I stored in the deep freeze. It's a D.I.Y. job. The only way to inseminate them is to catch them in season and I sit astride the rump facing her tail end. My weight is like the weight of the boar on her back so the sow stands still and I can put the semen filled straw into her vagina. This is my first inseminated litter!"

He paused and a wicked smile flitted across his face. "I suppose that you could call me the faither of this lot!"

Shortly after this incident we arranged a farmers' evening at the Angel Hotel. The speaker, supplied by one of the drug firms was going to talk on milking procedures on the modern dairy herd. After the audience was suitably mollified with refreshments the speaker, who was used to an audience in intensive dairying areas, commenced his talk. He pointed out that farmers should only spend four minutes milking each cow to avoid mastitis, and in a herring bone parlour could speed up the whole system without too much stress.

It all sounded so simple that very little could go wrong. During a slight pause a large hand was waved in the air. I felt a bit uneasy as the questioner was Joe Lane. "Yes Joe. Do you have a question?"

"Well yes!" responded Joe, beaming at the audience who knew him of old. "Maybe we're not as smart as the upcountry farmers or their cows, but from what I see the modern herdsman, with all the pressure of milking, has to be a cross between "a greyhound and an octeepoos!" There was complete silence before the room was gripped in thunderous applause.

A few weeks later I heard that Joe was walking into his piggery when he noticed a Landrover sitting in the drive with the bonnet raised and a figure bent over the engine. Recognising the figure he shouted "What be doing Treloar. Did somebody steal the engine?"

"I'd hope you would'n see me Joe but she came to an abrupt halt. I've been trying to adjust the carburettor but I cain't turn this bleddy old nut!"

After a couple of minutes assistance Joe continued "The problem is that the nut is too awkward to get at. The only solution would be to 'ave an eduucated ferret'.

Chapter Twenty-one

IN THE UNIVERSITY holidays I used to meet John Head and we got on extremely well when he 'saw practice' with us. We had both been involved in rugby and enjoyed a social pint along with a long-term aim to develop the small animal side of the practice. Charles had never worked with pets and John Saunders was temperamentally incapable of dealing with this aspect of practice.

At the end of August 1975 John Saunders and his family were preparing to go on holiday to London. On the morning of their departure I received an early morning call to say that John had died during the night. Of course this came as a great shock to everyone. It transpired that he had had a massive internal haemorrhage during the night and died without regaining consciousness. We could only be thankful that the family had not set off on their journey as undoubtedly he would have been travelling on the motorway at speeds in excess of 70 miles an hour.

After a short discussion we decided that, as the practice was booming, we must seek extra assistance. This was solved by the arrival of Tony Ross who eventually became a partner in 1985. About this time David and Hilary Cromey also joined the partnership. We then found ourselves with a practice of four partners and six assistants which indicated a healthy business. Charles Head and V had both retired and were delighted to take a back seat.

Anything can happen in this magic land of Cornwall. My colleagues were delighted when I mentioned that, after many night calls, I would be driving through Church Street in Helston and saw a large white rabbit sitting in the middle of the road. It always hopped up an alley and disappeared. Amongst the laughter this drew a number of comments such as drink, mad hatters and Alice in Wonderland. It was not until many years later that a neighbour by the name of Pascoe confessed that they kept several New Zealand White Giant bunnies who occasionally escaped in the night.

Stuart Williams, my erstwhile helper in the practice, was asked by Vera Head if he would like to plant some tulips in a small bed on the gravel path leading to the consulting rooms. "Yes! Mrs Head. I should like that as I can watch them growing."

Like a couple of expectant fathers we used to watch for the first green tips and then their growth until he had a dozen colourful tulips to delight the eye.

Stuart's lunch break was spent sitting inside the waiting room door soaking up the warmth of the noonday sun and almost dozing off. He was quietly meditating one beautiful day when he heard the scrunch of feet walking down the footpath. Silence followed and a woman's voice said, "My dear soul, look at they pretty flowers. We'll have a couple of they before we leave!"

For a couple of seconds Stuart was stunned as he considered that his pet tulips were being kidnapped. He quietly stuck his head around the entrance saying "Good afternoon my dears. Don't forget to take they with the greenfly on!"

Stuart was still very young and shy. One bright day a very rustic and somewhat unusual client brought in her cat "Foxy" for a check up. She and her husband lived a rather bohemian existence on the Lizard peninsula. "Can you have a look at 'Foxy,' Mr Stuart. I know he's getting on in years but he's started to look a bit moth eaten with several bare patches on his head."

"Mrs Mitchell," I commented. "Do you realise that from Helston down the Lizard peninsula we are finding numerous cases of ringworm. The reason I do not understand, but I suggest that you and your husband do a body check of each other in case you have any skin lesions."

There was a pregnant silence whilst she mulled over the situation and without any ceremony she dropped her trousers to her knees exposing a well developed pair of thighs. On one thigh there was a very large ringworm lesion. I heard a scrabbling behind me and glimpsed over my shoulder to see Stuart with his head in a cupboard feverishly arranging and rearranging the six bottles on the shelves. It was evident that he was suffering from too much information too early in life.

Steadying the rocking ship and sensing the impact of her actions, Mrs Mitchell restored her modesty whereupon Stuart came out of hibernation full of embarrassment. After she departed he commented drily "That lady should carry a government health warning!

Despite any failings, Stuart and I would go off and enjoy fishing together in the evening. As dusk dropped he would complain about the noise caused by the bats squeaking. It was only then that I realised that I had lost this ability to hear them as I grew older. "They're quite loud" continued Stuart. "Just like the sound of a beetle rubbing its elytra (wing covers) together." It was at this stage that I had to bow to his superior biological knowledge.

In the late seventies Charles realised that surgery was inevitable on his wounded leg This restricted his movements to four walls which he found to be very onerous, as he was essentially a 'people person'. Vtook him out in the car as much as possible to meet old friends, which was a great consolation. In 1981 he developed a cardiac condition and died. This was a cause of great sadness to his family but also to us who had worked with him. One of life's characters had passed away.

Life continued onwards and by 1986 both David and Tony had become partners. With four enthusiastic members the practice flourished so that we ended up with ten vets in our brand-new, custom-built premises on the Water-Ma-Trout industrial estate in Helston.

We had found the farming community to be so friendly and I ended up on the advisory committee of the Young Farmers Club. The YFC were so vibrant and full of ideas, and it gave me an excellent opportunity to mix with the members and their families. It was a very active club with activities ranging from sporting competitions to sheep-shearing and cookery.

Chapter Twenty-two

IT WAS A GLORIOUS 'blackbird morning', full of sunshine and the promise of an early spring. Long before breakfast my sleep was interrupted by a phone call from Tom Oliver, a semi-retired farmer who had spent much of his life with horses. "Oh! Mr Stuart, I'm some glad that it's you. We've just had a little filly born and she's wandering about like she can't see. Can you see her first thing."

This was a cry from the heart as he was panicking. "Right Tom, I shall be with you shortly. Make sure that she doesn't damage herself!"

I quickly dressed and was ready to depart when Alison our horsey daughter, who had jumped into bed with Margaret broke in "Can I come too Dad? I could help!"

We drove off to Roskorwell, across Goonhilly Downs in the glorious sunshine. All the time I was being interrogated by Alison about the filly's problem. My mind was awash with diagnoses. What could cause a foal to be blind? A hereditary condition, concussion or possibly a barker foal?

"I'm not sure Ali but she could be a 'Barker or dummy' foal if her blood and oxygen supply has been damaged. I've never seen one so we shall have to work it out".

We arrived at the paddock to a rather bemused mare wondering why her filly wouldn't suckle, and a confused foal with her head stuck in the hedge, wondering why the world was so dark.

The compelling evidence for this being a 'Barker" foal was before me. The mare had foaled whilst standing and the umbilical cord had broken as the foal hit the ground. The foal would be left with only half it's blood volume, the remainder was left in the placenta which now lay on the grass.

As soon as the foal staggered to its feet and followed the mare, it ran out of breath due to shortage of oxygen in the blood and was unable to see.

Tom muttered "I can't look after this little thing, Mr Stuart. Put her down for her sake."

"Be patient Tom," I replied. "Give her a chance. We shall find a way around this problem. I shall sedate her now and call back just before lunch."

On the way home Alison, as expected, was full of excitement and questions. "Can't we save her dad? She has had no time to live yet. I could come out every day and help her!" As we drove home I said to Ali. "Let's work out a plan. We could take the estate car back later later with a bale of straw. Then I'll persuade Tom to let us take her home for a few days.

"In the meantime we could prepare the garage as a loose box, bring in six bales of straw and bed her down. I will ask Johnny Walker the chemist for six containers of SMA baby food, and we must be prepared to feed the foal every two hours day and night for the next four days, and see if she gets her sight back." I was beginning to enjoy this adventure more than Ali.

We duly arrived back at lunchtime to find the foal relaxed but still blind. Tom did not need much persuading and was delighted to pass her over to our care. We drove back home with Ali and foal together in the back and dreams of the future very present.

I collected the SMA baby food and a few artificial cow's teats from Johnny Walker and we set down to the serious business of preparing her feeds. Of course the milk had to be at the correct temperature and the teat attached to a stout pop bottle. Of course Ali's horsey friend Tracey had to be in attendance, so I was assured that the patient was in good hands. The next problem was toileting with eager hands to shovel away the droppings.

There was no problem with two hourly feeds although a tad tiring and within forty-eight hours "Rilla" as she had been christened was able to see. By this time we had her fitted with a halter and lead rope which aided handling and I had decided that she should be exercised in the garden. This entailed carrying a moderately heavy foal down the steps and onto the garden.

We had to lunge Rilla on a long rein to exercise her and return her to some sort of normality. The patient improved in leaps and bounds whilst Ali and I grew more tired with feeding. As the pristine front lawn became more pock-marked with holes from little feet, I sensed a feeling of resistance from Margaret as her lawn began to resemble a golf course.

Eventually we decided that, after four days, Rilla was ready to back to her mother, if the mare would take her. We contacted Tom and headed back home to Roskorwell determined that Rilla should be put onto her mother to suckle. It worked and the foal was encouraged with me on the lead rope and Ali and Tracey holding hands around her bottom like a pair of rugby scrummagers pushing her towards the mare.

This became a twice-weekly ritual to take the girls to encourage Rilla to feed and make her halter broken. At the end of seven months came the time to wean Rilla and say goodbye, and the girls were very despondent. At this stage Tom gave the foal to Alison as a gift for all her hard work, and two very excited girls got together to plot the filly's future.

I had already laid down the ground rules 1) Ali must find pasture 2) She must work to provide fodder and 3) I did not intend to take her around the horse shows each weekend as Margaret and I must have a life of our own. Alison in her enthusiasm developed a tremendous work ethic and carried out her part of the bargain.

Alison would check up on Rilla every day. She had been loaned a paddock with a shelter in it. This also had space for fodder and as Rilla grew older the girls set to work breaking in this delightful character.

The time came when schooldays came to an end that she had to make a decision on

Rilla's future. I could not cope when she left for college so the she made the serious and very brave decision to sell her to a good home as she wished to use the proceeds to the travel through N. America and see her relatives. This was a turning point in her life!

At this time I had the opportunity to fulfil my dream of studying fish medicine; applied for and was accepted for an aquatic pathobiology course in Stirling. This was a great leap into the unknown, as Margaret and I had never been separated before.

I departed for Stirling early in September, full of doubts as to whether I was doing the right thing by my family. I had my partners' blessings as long as I paid for a locum, and Margaret, in her wisdom, realised that after 22 years in practice that I needed a new challenge.

Despite all the doubts my children had the answer to our quandary and regaled all and sundry with "Dad's going to college two weeks before Donal and Alison which leaves mum at home to guide Kate through her school leaving year!"

My first few weeks at Stirling University were an eye opener. I was living on the fourth floor of a concrete block with a wonderful view of the students collecting plant samples from the lawns. I was wrong: they were hunting for magic mushrooms to feed their habit!

Life had changed in the intervening years. Students had money which made life much easier. They could afford to drink, drive and could become involved in politics and free love.

I was the grandaddy of the MSc course, who were a mixed bunch from across the globe, and included many who came from third world countries to learn fish farming techniques. My greatest challenge was to re-educate myself to study after so many years, and this took six weeks of concentration when I worked until the small hours of the morning. To balance out my life I took up squash, snorkelling and dancing to put life and mettle in my heels.

In such a lovely campus I would walk down to one of the Lochans each morning in the hope of catching a trout for breakfast. Pressure of work was such that I had little spare time to go off campus for my entertainment.

I found the whole mix of students at the university to be a fascinating insight into youth. They varied in age from sixteen years old to septuagenarians. They were much more affluent than in my university days but curiously they had more problems with their freedom.

The cloistered life suited my intent to pursue the course as I encountered subjects such as electron microscopy and calculus which were new to me. The commercial fish farm visits were an eye-opener as as these were new experiences and I was surprised to find many men with doctorates cleaning out the tanks to make a living. Acquiring a Ph.D. indicates that you have concentrated your studies so narrowly that you can become almost unemployable in the commercial field.

The year flew past and I left Stirling in May to write my thesis back at home. Margaret and I were so delighted to be reunited and she helped me to put in many hours work by editing my thesis. When I did eventually re-start work in the practice I was completely rejuvenated and enjoying the farm work.

I was involved increasingly in more fish medicine as there were numerous small fish farms in the area, and my interest spread. I had numerous calls from people with pond and aquarium fish. I had not realised how involved people became with their fish and the money they spent on acquiring pond fish. Koi carp were high on the payment scale and have been known to command a million dollars.

Eventually most of the fish farms closed down except one which asked me to act as unpaid advisor. I had great fun watching this farm develop as I could not have become a partner whilst I was in veterinary practice. The owners struggled for several years, until one day they announced that they had gone into receivership. I was very sympathetic until the Midland Bank sent me a bill for £380,000 as I was the only solvent partner.

This was a great shock as I had informed my wife, my partners, the bank manager and my accountant that I did not intend to become a partner in the fishery. I became very depressed until my solicitor and accountant asked to see the partnership agreement. The lack of response from the bank ended the problem. It appeared that the manager had been careless enough to permit a vast debt to develop without security. Before I could talk to him he was mysteriously transferred away to Somerset.

John Lawrance farmed at Gweleath in Cury with his son. They ran a very efficient dairy unit but for the past few months they had had a continuous problem with mastitis.

Every time that we cured the condition it would recur. Eventually we sought help from the government veterinary laboratory in Truro, but in vain. The assistance extended to the regional laboratory in in Bristol and then to the Central Veterinary centre in Surrey. Many wise men pondered and stroked their beards without success. We were at our wits end until one day John turned to me and said, "Look, I have read in the Farmer's Weekly that a homoeopathic vet up country has been successfully treating a similar problem. Can we ask him for a second opinion? "

I was delighted as we were getting nowhere with conventional medicine and offered to contact Chris Day, the vet in question, as I had always leaned towards the unconventional, if in doubt!

We took Chris to the farm and produced bacteriology reports from the laboratories. He examined the premises and cattle. He questioned us about water supplies to the premises and use of a water trough for the cattle.

Within a week the medication arrived with instructions to add five ml. regularly to the water trough. This appeared to be an extremely unreal way to treat a herd but we should persevere. John's uncle had also paid a visit and demonstrated that two ley lines actually met in the cow cubicles where the cattle remained at night, and that such an occurrence could cause problems.

The whole condition cleared up within a month and I was determined to investigate homoeopathy in greater depth as this could be yet another tool in our fight against disease.

I found out that homeopathic courses were held at regular intervals at The Royal Homeopathic Hospital in London and I booked in to attend a series. The first course that I attended completely confused me as the basic concept of homeopathy is contrary to much of my formal teaching at college.

Many of my more intelligent colleagues cannot grasp the cult of using minimal doses. Are they channelled into a narrow field of thought and unable to think out of the box? They regard homeopathy as occult instead of studying the subject.

I have had many applications of this type of medicine and still use it.

In addition to my homeopathic interests I found that I was of necessity becoming involved in dowsing and ley lines. Along with ley lines and magnetic lines of force I began to understand how animals migrate, how aborigines go walkabout and Bushmen in the Kalahari can disappear and return at an appointed time. There is so much that we do not understand!

As time went on I became more and more involved in fish medicine -goldfish and carp appeared from many miles away. With the blessing of my colleagues I used more and more homoeopathy in large and small animal practice. It was a very economic means of medication and I made a point of giving my clients the choice of traditional or homeopathic treatments.

And in conclusion....

THE FAMILY HAD ALL flown the nest for places as far flung as Mongolia, Hong Kong and New Zealand so we have travelled across the world in alternate years to visit our children and enjoy the company of Alison's extended family.

I was asked to give a talk at Truro hospital one evening when my generous hosts offered me a glass of wine. As I accepted I felt a severe pain in my chest which appeared to oscillate from left to right. Immediately the vision of a magazine article on heart attacks, which I had read, flashed through my mind. I heard myself in a detached manner say "Thank you but I'm having a heart attack so could you order me a doctor whilst I go and lie down"

Realising that it was critical not to panic I searched my mind for a sense of tranquility in order to relax. Then it came to me that I could be a goldfish being gently wafted around in a tidal wave. To the uninitiated this may seem eccentric but that little fish helped me through a sticky patch until the nurse and doctor arrived.

Donal, arrived shortly afterwards with Margaret. He was very shaken and pale but Margaret was as calm and serene as ever-my rock! Her appearance steadied any doubts that I might have had on my condition. The medical care was first rate and I was home within ten days.

At this stage my partners banned me from night duties and insisted that I slowed down. This was the stage in my life when my old ailments such as slipped discs and general assault from farm animals started to take its toll. I was unable to stand for long periods and gradually cut down my working hours until I retired in 1994, retaining my consultancies in homoeopathy and fish diseases.

Retirement has sealed a bond in life so that we can travel to New Zealand and I can pursue my joy of writing about our life together!